RIPPLES
FROM THE EDGE OF LIFE

ROLAND CHESTERS

D1471058

SilverWood

Published in 2018 by SilverWood Books

SilverWood Books Ltd
14 Small Street, Bristol, BS1 1DE, United Kingdom
www.silverwoodbooks.co.uk

ISBN 978-1-78132-709-8 (paperback)
ISBN 978-1-78132-710-4 (ebook)

British Library Cataloguing in Publication Data
A CIP catalogue record for this book is available from the British Library

Page design and typesetting by SilverWood Books
Printed on responsibly sourced paper

CONTENTS

ACKNOWLEDGEMENTS

This book would not exist without the input of the many contributors.

I must therefore thank those people who agreed to put on record their recollection of how it felt to be a part of my journey through a HIV/AIDS diagnosis: Alli, Anne, David, Dean, Esther, Joyce, Kate, Maddy, Marta, Mary, Pip and Suzanne.

My thanks also go to those who volunteered to share their narrative: Andy, Chris, Esther, Danny, Florence, Chris, Jimmy, Kevin, Maurice, Ruth, Simon, Steve and Steven.

Tom has kept me on the straight and narrow (well, somewhat straight) and his expert advice has been invaluable.

My final thanks must go to the man who has been my rock and my pillow, who has been on every step of this journey with me, who never asked or wanted to but has been unstinting in his love and support: Richard.

FOREWORD

IAN GREEN, CEO, TERRENCE HIGGINS TRUST

I have known Roland for a number of years now and have always enjoyed our conversations. When he asked if I would be prepared to write a foreword to his book I immediately said yes, because I knew that Roland would write with sensitivity, good grace and humour, whilst not glossing over some of the challenges that he has faced in his journey. What I was not expecting, however, was to be so moved by what I read, particularly as someone who has lived with HIV myself for over twenty years. It enabled me to reflect on my own experiences and journey.

Not long after the HIV and AIDS epidemic hit the UK, the Government introduced the infamous 'tombstone' adverts, which caused people across the country to fear the virus. And fear those who had it.

The fear instilled by these adverts inspired a relentless scare-mongering campaign among tabloid media, which served only to solidify the stigma surrounding the virus and further isolate people living with HIV. Many of these people were already from minority backgrounds, such as gay and bi-sexual men, black African people or members of the trans community, and for them this stigma man-ifested in a doubly damaging form of dual discrimination.

Such was the unwavering influence of tabloid reporting on HIV coupled with the tombstone adverts that, despite enormous medical advances over the decades that followed, fear, stigma and discrimination still continue to consume the lives of many people living with HIV today.

One man who experienced this discrimination was Terry Higgins, who lost his life to HIV in 1982.

In response to his death and the mistreatment faced by others like him, Terry's friends formed the Terrence Higgins Trust in his name, to humanise how HIV is seen in the UK and help better the lives of people living with the virus.

Since then we have seen great medical advances and, in 1996, effective treatment for HIV first became available.

The treatment reduces the HIV virus in the bloodstream until the amount left is what's called 'undetectable'. That means that those on effective treatment, and so are undetectable, can live long and healthy lives.

This great news means that we're now seeing the first generation to live with HIV into old age and, moving forward, we must ensure that we are best set to support our ageing HIV population.

In addition to advances in treatment came the PARTNER study, which has scientifically proven that people living with HIV and who are on effective treatment cannot pass it on.

While not a cure, this does mean that people living with HIV and who are on effective treatment are able to date, start a family and enjoy a healthy sex life without fear of passing on the virus.

Testing for HIV has also come on leaps and bounds. We've come a long way since the 1980s, where I remember waiting up to three weeks for test results, for which I'd used a false name to retrieve because of the stigma I felt and faced at the time.

Today, charities like Terrence Higgins Trust test people proudly and publicly in community settings, supermarkets, churches and, in 2016, at a colourful pop-up shop in east London. We now also have access to self-test kits, which enable those who would rather not test in public to do so privately and at home instead.

Despite the leaps and bounds in treatment and testing however, there has been very little shift in attitudes toward HIV and people who are living with it.

While people living with HIV might be protected in law under the Equality Act 2010, meaning it is illegal to discriminate against someone with HIV in employment, health care or access to goods and services because of their status, stigma still very much exists.

We still hear countless experiences of discrimination against people living with HIV that many would think were from the 1980s and not from 2018.

For instance, one in four Britons still thinks that sharing a toothbrush can cause HIV transmission. And one in five believe that HIV can be transmitted through kissing.

This kind of stigma sticks, and can have a huge impact on the mental health of people living with HIV, their relationships and their sense of self.

It can also discourage people from being tested for HIV, or can cause them to delay getting tested. This may lead to late diagnoses, unwitting transmission or people continuing to live with HIV while being unaware of it.

One in seven people living with HIV don't know that they have it and, in order to end HIV transmission, it's vital that people test regularly and know how to best use the combination of prevention tools available to them.

We can't achieve this unless young people learn about HIV and sexual health as part of inclusive Relationships and Sex Education, and are equipped with the knowledge to best practice safe sex when the time comes.

Testing for HIV must also become much more routine and should be seen as no different to visiting a dentist or having your blood pressure taken.

To achieve this, and to continue combatting stigma and busting myths surrounding the virus, we must also continue amplifying the voices of people living with HIV in the UK.

We're grateful to all of those people who allow us to share their stories, and to the supportive allies who help these stories reach far and wide, including our volunteers and donors, corporate partners, supportive journalists or other close friends of Terrence Higgins Trust.

One of those friends is Prince Harry, who spent the morning with the Terrence Higgins Trust during National HIV Testing Week in 2017, learning about self-test kits and the importance of knowing your status.

Two weeks later, he and Meghan Markle then joined us at our World AIDS Day event in Nottingham, talking to people living with HIV and hearing from local groups about how they support those who are HIV positive.

This kind of work is invaluable and, like the support given by the late, wonderful Princess Diana to people with HIV and AIDS in the 1980s, really helps to tackle stigma at an international level.

It also demonstrates the fact that each and every one of us has a part to play in the fight to end HIV transmission in the UK and the stigma that surrounds it.

This wonderful book, *Ripples,* highlights the hurdles and hardship that people diagnosed with HIV so often come up against.

Roland's story, and so many of the others which he shares in his book, truly demonstrate the power of courage, love and determination, which are often needed to overcome those hurdles, but also to look positively to the future – a future without fear, discrimination and stigma. He starts the book by saying that he is no author – I disagree. He tells his story with honesty and passion and the book deserves to be widely read.

We've come a long way over the last thirty years to fight the HIV epidemic and end the stigma surrounding the virus, but there still remains much more work to do.

As Roland so powerfully states in the book

> Life isn't about being afraid of the thunderstorms. It's about learning how to dance in the rain. There have been quite a few thunderstorms in my life and each time, I got out there and danced, each time learning new steps and a different rhythm. There will undoubtedly be more thunderstorms ahead. So if you see me out there, dancing in the rain, please come and join me. There is nothing worse than dancing alone.

I, for one, am dancing with you, Roland.

From all us living with HIV thank you for so powerfully sharing your story and for demonstrating page by page, courage, love, determination and hopefulness.

INTRODUCTION

Ripple: a particular feeling or effect that spreads through someone or something – *Oxford English Dictionary*

I am not an author. This will not be the first in a series of volumes to match *War and Peace* (although as themes those could be quite pertinent to the contents of this publication!). I have no literary ambitions. What I do have is a need to tell my story. Not because it is in any way unique or special, but because I think that it is potentially representative of the current state of HIV/AIDS in the UK and because there is so little else published on this topic. I hope that this one, small piece of work, encompassing not just my voice, but those affected by my 'ripple' and others who are also living with this condition, will help to cast a light into its murky shadows. Too long – and still – highly stigmatised, there is a need for those of us who are able, to stand up and be counted.

Once a ripple has been set in motion it is unstoppable. The impact of a traumatic diagnosis, not just of HIV but of any life-changing illness, not only on the individual but also on those that surround them cannot be under estimated. The consequences of that ripple can be unforeseen and unexpected.

If the ripples in this book reach you, move you, educate, inspire or challenge you, then my job has been done.

PROLOGUE

I stared out of the carriage window as the 17.53 from Waterloo rattled towards Surbiton, the grimy sprawl of south London rapidly giving way to the leafier parts of Surrey. I could almost set my watch to the time we passed certain landmarks: shops, offices, houses, stations, parks. It was all so familiar; so horribly, boringly familiar and I felt drained and exhausted with it all.

Thank goodness, then, that from tomorrow I had a two-week holiday in the Italian Lakes to look forward to. I knew that by the time I arrived home Richard, my partner, would have packed the bags, printed the tickets and unearthed the passports. All I had to do was turn up, which was just as well because I was capable of little else.

For months and months I'd felt unwell. Nausea, poor balance and coordination, loss of control over arm and leg movements, tetchiness, extreme exhaustion and incoherent speech were all part of my daily life. I'd had test after test, and scan after scan, with no clear diagnosis of what was wrong with me. Whatever it might be, it was tearing my body and mind apart – but what was it? No one seemed to know. I just had to get on with it.

The day before I'd had an HIV test on the recommendation of

a respiratory specialist who'd been examining my lungs for nodules (which turned out to be nothing more scary than chickenpox scars). It was about the only test I hadn't had – and the one I felt was the least necessary. Yes, I'm gay but had never been involved in promiscuity or risky sex of any kind, having had just two long-term partners. But if an HIV test could rule *that* out as well, it was worth doing.

I arrived home to find my mother and brother being attended to by Richard. My mother adored Richard and because she lived close by she would frequently call on us, particularly if we were going away. We chatted, and once they finished their coffee they made moves to go, wishing us a good holiday.

After the front door had clicked to I went into the bedroom, expecting to find everything I needed for the holiday ready and waiting. Except this time, there were no clothes on the bed to pack, and no suitcase in which to pack them. I went into the living room, where Richard was sitting in silence.

"Er, don't you think we ought to start packing?" I said. "If we leave it any longer we'll end up in a panic."

In response, Richard beckoned me to the sofa and pointed to the seat next to him. Puzzled, I sat down. Then he hugged me and started to cry. I was shocked. He's a big, strong man, physically and mentally, and not given to floods of tears. What on earth was going on?

"What is it?" I asked. "What's happened? Is it serious? Is it bad news from home?"

Richard's family are thousands of miles away, in Barbados. But he shook his head. It wasn't them.

"It's us," he sobbed. "We aren't going away, Roland. We can't. I'm so sorry."

"Why? Why can't we?"

"The specialist rang. The one who did the test yesterday. He wanted your office number, because…"

"Because what!?"

"Because he said that we can't go away. The test result came back. Roland, you're positive. HIV positive. You're really ill. We can't go to Italy. If we do...you won't come home alive. It's that bad. I'm so, so sorry."

PART ONE

CHAPTER ONE

Two weeks to live. That was the prognosis. Unless someone, somewhere, acted fast I would be dead in just fourteen days. I was so ill and exhausted that I could barely take it in. I just wanted to sleep. Perhaps I just wanted to die, putting an end to the sheer weariness I'd been experiencing. Life changing as it was, at that point it seemed just another 'thing' to contend with. As I sunk my face into the pillow and hoped for oblivion, temporary or otherwise, my only thought was, 'Well at least I know now.'

For the previous two years I'd worked at the Foreign and Commonwealth Office (FCO) in central London as a language-testing specialist. The FCO provides tuition for officers who will be serving overseas to a level of language required to do their job when they arrive. They receive the tuition and are tested on it, and I supervised those tests. By any standard it was a good job. I managed a team of five people in an interesting, challenging and varied environment. I got to travel, and to meet people from across the world. I shouldn't have been feeling so downhearted, deflated and totally exhausted, mentally and physically. So why was I?

Before my diagnosis, the answer to this seemed obvious to me: a mid-life crisis. I was in my mid-forties, the somewhat dangerous period at which a man begins to ask himself the big questions in life.

'Who am I?' 'Why am I here?' 'What have I achieved?' 'What have I done?' 'What do I regret not doing?' All those, and more, pointed to that inescapable conclusion. Not being one to naturally swap my inner turmoil for a shiny new Harley Davidson or a string of girlfriends (or in my case, boyfriends) I kept these thoughts mainly to myself. If it really was the fabled 'male-menopause' then surely it would pass without the need for extensive tattooing or time in a Buddhist monastery.

Unfortunately, I was increasingly unable to hide the physical symptoms of whatever was going on internally. During my previous two years at the FCO I'd been temporarily promoted to cover my line manager's duties for six months while she was off sick. It was highly pressurised and although I coped with it reasonably well, her return to work prompted a period in which I became unresponsive and ineffective. I started to fall asleep at my desk for no apparent reason. Employers don't like it when you do that too often. I can't think why. In addition, the commute home to Surbiton was increasingly fraught with confusion. I'd get off a train, phone Richard and say, "I don't know where I am."

"Look at the station sign," he'd reply, "and tell me what it says. Then I'll come to pick you up." He'd collect me in Chessington, or Tolworth, or Woking, and I'd have no explanation as to why I'd ended up there. I hadn't fallen asleep on the train; I'd simply got on the wrong one. Commuter trains were usually packed, with no seats available and I was having problems standing and balancing. Fellow commuters might have thought I was drunk – but I don't drink! Richard then started to drive me to Wimbledon in the mornings, so that I could take the Tube into work because I could guarantee that at least that way I would get a seat.

The days dragged by in a haze of weariness, exhaustion and bad temper. I began to get niggly with staff at work for no great reason other than my own intolerance. Yet normally I wasn't that sort of person. Sure, I have my quirks, foibles and idiosyncrasies like anyone else. But intolerance? Not me…

Also 'not me' was the feeling of losing my balance and coordination. I'm not afraid to admit that I'm not the world's greatest sportsman. But finding difficulty in just walking? Almost falling over when crossing roads? My handwriting, of which I had always been proud, was now a succession of messy squiggles that even I had problems deciphering. And not being able to speak clearly, too. I've always had clear diction and now people would say, "Roland, you're mumbling, speak up. We can't understand what you're saying…"

I sometimes indulge in a little bit of amateur dramatics. I had a relatively minor role in a period drama but I was having difficulty remembering the lines – not something that had been an issue for me before. The director of the play assigned someone to me to help me learn the lines. I was mortified.

It was driving me mad, to the point where I genuinely wondered if I was going mad. The confusion, the ill-temper, the lack of coordination… It was enough for me to fear for my sanity. Richard, as ever, was pragmatic and practical.

"You're not going mad," he said, "but there's obviously something wrong. You're just not…you. For God's sake, go and see the GP. At least it's a start."

I've never been an 'ill person'. I'm not constantly banging on the doctor's door, demanding that all manner of things be checked out. But something was clearly wrong, and so we began a trail of medical examinations by various specialists; heart scans, diets, 'health action plans' and positive thinking that led…well, nowhere at all. The scans proved nothing, and my heart was fine. By this time I'd developed the most agonising pains in my head, blinding bursts of white heat that would last only for a few seconds but felt crippling when they attacked. There was something wrong, and someone needed to tell me what it was.

At the time, Richard was working for a company that as a perk offered private healthcare to employees and their partners. He made enquiries and discovered there was a neurologist in Harley Street who could see me under the terms of the healthcare cover. Well, it was worth a try and if a Harley Street doctor can't tell you what's the matter, who can? An appointment was made and in February 2006 I attended the neurologist's clinic. He inspected me thoroughly before concluding that I had 'ice-pick syndrome'. I asked what this might be.

"They're called ice-pick pains because they feel as though someone is stabbing an ice-pick into your head," he said, describing exactly what was going on inside my skull. "They're common in patients with a personal or family history of migraine." I'd told him that, while I'd never suffered from migraine, my mother had.

"Is there anything that can be done for them?" I asked.

"They are benign," he replied, "but they're very difficult to treat with painkillers. I'm afraid you'll just have to put up with them and see if they go away. Oh, and I should have asked…are you depressed?"

"I'm hardly cheerful," I said, "and why would I be? I'm sure it's because of all the pain and the difficulties I'm having."

"Hmm," he said, "I think we should try you on a course of anti-depressants. See how you do on those."

Some days later a report arrived with my GP. As he mentioned, the neurologist diagnosed 'ice-pick syndrome' but could find no other 'significant abnormalities' apart from some discomfort on my neck. However, I was prescribed a dose of Citalopram, an anti-depressant. I didn't even bother to cash in the prescription.

I was terribly confused at the time. The neurologist had identified something, but 'ice-pick pains' sounded very vague and were seemingly untreatable. I just wanted someone to say, 'this is what is happening, this is how to make it better'. But no one had, and it seemed that no one ever would. The headaches, the wrong trains and the lack of coordination carried on unabated. And so did the problems at work. In March I received a mid-term performance and development review, of the kind that only the Civil Service can deliver in all its bureaucratic glory. I was praised for my 'commitment and ability to establish procedures' and a 'calm approach to problems'. However, there was one telling paragraph:

"During some periods, Roland suffered some problems with concentration and delivery at his usual speed. This was openly discussed, as at some stage this was noticed outside our department and came across as lack of interest and loss of motivation. His colleagues also discretely mentioned their concerns about Roland's well-being."

So the message was clear: 'Roland is not pulling his weight, and it is being noticed in the department.' I had no explanation for it, other than I felt dreadfully unwell – and I had no explanation for that either. And I was starting to feel scared. How much longer could I go on like this?

Richard, in his wisdom and kindness, could see I needed a break and a rest. And where better for me than Paris? My mother was French, from Paris, and we'd made many visits there as a family. I'd also lived, and was partly educated, there so the city was as familiar to me as London. It had no associations with stressful work or commuting or feeling lousy. A weekend away was just what I needed – or so we thought.

*

Within twenty-four hours of arriving, I was on the way home again. We were on the Metro, heading for Montmartre, when I keeled over and collapsed. Richard had to drag me up the Metro steps and out into the street, where I kind of came to and was just about fit enough to make it back to the hotel. Richard packed our bags for the sorry journey to the Gare Du Nord and home. The following weekend we went to stay with friends on the Isle of Wight who are keen walkers. We were walking up a hill and I couldn't make it. They thought I was having a heart attack and one of our friends had to go and get their car so they could get me home. I remember hardly anything of either weekend, but both incidents were enough to convince Richard that he ought to accompany me to further medical appointments so that he could ask for explanations and challenge any more vague attempts to define what was wrong with me. At that stage, I simply didn't have the energy to fight for my own well-being.

One of these appointments was on 31 August 2006, at Kingston Hospital with a respiratory consultant, relating to a worrying series of nodules found on my lungs during a heart scan. Richard came with me and I introduced him as my partner. The specialist quickly disabused me of the idea that I might have lung cancer. I'd never been a smoker and it was thought, even before an MRI scan, that they were benign. As it turned out, they were chickenpox scars from childhood, so at least cancer could be ruled out as a diagnosis for my on-going problems.

The doctor was a sympathetic man and recognised that we were a same-sex couple. He listened carefully as I described my symptoms. "It's a puzzle," he said, "and by your notes I can see that you've been tested for all sorts of things. Do you mind if I ask if you've ever been tested for HIV?"

Momentarily I was taken aback. "No," I said, "I've never been tested for that. I've never felt it necessary, to be honest."

This was true. I'd never been what you might described as a 'scene' gay man, preferring an evening at the opera to a sweaty night in a club pumping out electro disco. I was openly gay, but I never wore it as a badge. My sexuality didn't define me; it was just part of who I was, and it still is. I'd been single for some years before entering into two long-term monogamous relationships, one with Graham and the other with Richard that, by then, had lasted a decade. Richard and I volunteered for the Food Chain, delivering meals to isolated people with HIV, so I knew the impact it had on lives and the devastation it could cause. But I didn't for a minute think that I was THAT closely associated with the disease.

"So would you be interested in taking a test?" the doctor asked.

"I'm not sure it's going to prove anything," I said, "but I've been tested for everything else and I still don't know what the problem is. So let's do the test. Test me for anything."

So he did. It was such a simple matter that it hardly bears description here. Blood was taken, sent off somewhere, and that was it. During the course of the test I mentioned that Richard and I had booked a fortnight's holiday to the Italian Lakes beginning on Saturday. After the Paris debacle I was hoping that I'd finally manage to relax without falling in a heap somewhere. The holiday was for Richard's benefit too, as he'd just been made redundant and needed some time to regroup and think about what he'd like to do next. Picking up the results of the HIV test the following day was just another inconvenience in what was likely to be a busy Friday packing and preparing for Italy, so I told the specialist I'd collect them after the holiday.

The following day I crawled into work following the usual uncomfortable game of sardines on the Surbiton to Waterloo train. 'Only one day to go,' I kept telling myself, 'only one more day to go.'

By the end of the day it was all over and I made my weary way home looking forward to two weeks' break by the water and with the most stunning views of the surrounding mountains. If this didn't sort me out, or at least give me some temporary respite, I didn't know what would. Little did I know that Richard had already received the phone call that would explode a bomb in both our lives.

CHAPTER TWO

It's fair to say (and although I admit I haven't checked, I don't feel it's really necessary) that my mother is probably the only born and bred Parisian ever to have swapped the 'City of Light' for an insular industrial town in the north-west of England not noted for its colour, its sense of wonder or its Bohemian ways.

Accrington was that place; a cotton mill and brick-making town past its best, even in the early 1950s. Aside from the comedic name of its football team (Accrington Stanley), the town is probably best known for the appalling casualties its 'Pals' battalion suffered on 1 July 1916 – the first day of the Battle of the Somme. Hardly a place of light and joy then, but when you're in love it's not where your heart is physically, it is who it belongs to – and in this case her heart belonged very much to my father.

He was from Stockport and was training to be a civil engineer when he met my mother aboard a pleasure boat on the Thames. Having suffered many deprivations in occupied France during the war she was discovering a new sense of freedom and was on a European grand tour. London was one of her first stops and it was there she met my father. It seemed to be love at first sight and, Accrington notwithstanding, she married him and went to live with him up north where he was working for the English Electric

Company, located just outside the East Lancashire town.

Mum was one of identical girl twins. When they were born their parents weren't expecting two and had only thought of one name: Claudine. When my grandfather went to register their births they hadn't had time to think of another name and, caught on the spot, he put down the second name as Claudie. And that was that, separated by one consonant, my mother was Claudie, my aunt, Claudine. They were so similar that, as the threat of a German invasion loomed and my grandmother decided it could potentially be useful for her girls to be able to communicate in German but could not afford for them both to have private lessons, they attended on alternate weeks. The tutor never cottoned on that he was seeing two different children, but couldn't quite understand why they weren't making as much progress as he would have anticipated! They were fourteen when war was declared and evacuated from Paris a number of times. The last time, they fled to my great-grandparents in Normandy (in hindsight, not the best of ideas!).

However, they had been separated from their father. He was a carpenter working for the city of Paris and had been taken by the Germans to dig graves in the Bois de Boulogne for patriots who had been shot by the invading forces. He heard that twins had been killed on the street where they lived during a bombing raid, so he escaped, found that his family had left the city, stole a bike and followed them. My mother, aunt, their older sister and my grandmother had hitched a lift on an open cattle truck, along with many others fleeing the capital. German planes strafed them and they jumped out to hide under the trucks. In so doing my mother and aunt lost their shoes and continued literally on foot. When my grandfather eventually caught up with them he decided to make them a pair of wooden clogs each to help with the walking. But he was a carpenter, not a clog maker and by the time my mum and aunt arrived in Normandy all the small bones in their feet were broken. They both had hideously deformed feet for the rest of their lives – a source of great discomfort, both real and psychological, as they both loved shoes.

In the immediate post-war years mum suffered severe depression. It was only after she died, when our family GP was sent her French medical records, that Philip and I discovered that she had been subjected to electro-shock treatment at that time. She never spoke about it. I was saddened, but not surprised, to find out about it.

I never knew either grandfather. My paternal grandmother was a very typical English lady of her generation, with a set routine of laundry on Monday, baking on Tuesday, etc. She loved to bake and whenever we visited there were always freshly made cakes, biscuits and other goodies, which my gran would pack into a tin for us to take home. It was only many years after she died, in her mid-eighties, that I discovered she had had a full mastectomy when in her mid-twenties. This must have been early in the twentieth century and I suspect a radical and dangerous procedure at that time.

My maternal grandmother was a devout Catholic. During the war she had supported a local priest in secretly arranging marriages between Jewish and gentile couples so that the Jewish partner could evade being rounded up and taken away. In later years she opted to go into retreat into a convent so that she would not be a burden to her family. While there, she had all her teeth removed, believing that the suffering she would endure as a result of this would give her direct access to a better afterlife. I hope that, for her sake, this proved to be true.

My dad, Peter, was an only child. A tall, blond, good-looking youth, but shy and introverted. Mum was a more of a glamorous Hollywood starlet – and definitely not shy! I don't think the poor man stood a chance once she had set her cap at him. I think he was fascinated and bemused by her and was happy to be in the shadow of the brilliant Parisian light she cast around her. When he told his parents that he had become engaged to a Parisian woman they were, apparently, initially horrified. Pictures of French floozies obviously sped through their minds, but once they had met Claudie they too were completely bowled over. When my mother died we found love letters my father had written to her while they were engaged, when she was still in Paris and he was in London. I didn't read too many of them, it was too intrusive, but theirs was clearly a passionate and loving relationship.

They were married in Stockport, Claudie's father giving her away. He spoke no English and was a deeply shy man, but Peter had written the 'Father of the Bride' speech for him in English and had coached him in how to deliver it. As he was about to give away his daughter, he took her to one side and reminded her that it was not too late to change her mind if she decided she couldn't live in a country where they couldn't even make decent coffee!

I admire tremendously my mother's courage. To leave one's homeland and family, to travel to a relatively unknown country with only a little command of the language and set up one's own family far away from the bright lights of an exotic European capital, is no mean feat. She had to renounce her Catholicism (no great hardship for her) and her nationality in order to marry. I can only applaud her bravery and resolution in doing so.

My brother arrived first, in 1957, and I came along two and a half years later, in 1959. Mother had spoken French to Philip, my brother, up to the age he started school, and at that point his English was underpinned by a French accent. One day, though, he came home and asked my mother why she couldn't talk like all the other mums picking up their children from school. Mother took the point; Accrington was hardly cosmopolitan and the word 'multiculturalism' hadn't even been invented, so we became a family of English-only speakers, mother included.

That said, when I was about three, dad was asked to go and do some work in Germany for an extended period. He didn't want to leave his family behind but mum was concerned about exposing Philip and me to any German influences at such a young and tender age. So we were left in our aunt's care in Paris while our parents went to Germany. On their return to Paris a few months later, my mum found that I was calling my aunt 'maman'! Well, they were identical, but suffice it to say that that never happened again.

My mother was a sociable woman and she threw herself into Accrington life, taking on a number of jobs including teaching French at the primary school I attended. She would travel to Paris alone for a holiday every year and when she came home my father was overjoyed to see her, assuming (possibly with some justification) that one day she might never return. Otherwise, he was a rather Victorian father with a lower case 'v'. He wasn't draconian or unkind or overbearing; he was simply somewhat distant and unemotional, like a lot of fathers of that era. Their fathers and grandfathers had been the same and they saw no reason to change the status quo. He was also shy and self-effacing, and didn't cope well with stress. He was made redundant when I was about eleven and again a few years later and although he picked up other jobs, the demise of heavy engineering in the north of England meant that joblessness was always a threat. Father's way of coping was to internalise everything and he was a heavy smoker, too. Sadly, the writing was on the wall for him.

We had a relatively uneventful childhood. While other families in our street were large, noisy and extended, ours was small and quiet. I was quite the petite child up until the age of about eight or nine, when I suddenly and inexplicably ballooned in weight. I remember visits to Accrington Victoria Hospital so that doctors could take blood tests at different times, including at midnight. Given my weight issue, the cakes and biscuits my paternal grandmother baked for us to take home after we'd visited her were donated to the birds which gathered knowingly on our lawn – much to the chagrin of my brother and father! No one ever seemed able to work out what my weight problem was caused by and so I trundled on through childhood, enjoying music and languages and detesting sport and anything competitive. I did once join the Boy Scouts, but only because I rather admired the neckerchief and woggle they wore. Once I'd obtained those, I left.

"Ah!" you might say. "Hates sport, likes classical music, has an eye for fashion. I think I know where this is heading…" Well, you might do, but I certainly didn't, not even when my father returned from a business trip to Italy and brought my brother and me an Action Man each. These were much coveted because at the time they weren't on sale in the UK. Philip immediately took his off to play war, while I made a collection of nice little outfits for mine. Today, more enlightened parents might understand what was going on with their sensitive son but in those days being gay wasn't something one bandied around in public, least of all in Accrington.

However, I certainly wasn't the only 'gay in the town'. Occasionally, when people find out where I'm from, I'm asked if I knew Jeanette Winterson, the novelist and lesbian activist who grew up in Accrington and wrote the acclaimed *Oranges Are Not The Only Fruit*, about growing up with her adoptive parents, particularly her fiercely religious mother. The answer is that 'yes', I did know her. Her adoptive grandparents lived next door to us and as children of the same age, we regularly played together. With her, I even attended the Elim Pentecostal Church a couple of times where the kind of fire-brand preaching outlined in her book was regularly heard. I didn't really know anything about the difficulties she was experiencing at home and we drifted apart in our teens and lost touch. However, when 'Oranges' was published in the mid-1980s I went to see her at the British Film Institute viewing of the television series.

"Hi Jeanette!" I said. "Remember me? Roland...from Accrington?"

"Hmm," she replied, looking at me askance. Disappointed, I walked away. Perhaps she didn't want any uncomfortable reminders of a past she'd left behind. And I don't blame her.

The other 'gay in the town' whom I didn't know, but wish I had, was Mike Jackson, who set up Lesbians and Gays Support the Miners during the 1984–85 dispute, and whose story was featured in the 2014 hit British film *Pride*. Mike and his band of gay and lesbian activists, marginalised at the height of the AIDS epidemic, decamp to south Wales where they meet and bond with striking miners and their families. The film is incredibly heart-warming and moving, and although Mike is five years older than me (and therefore I never knew him) it's good to know that someone else trying to make a difference is from the same town.

I was obviously 'different' at school (my form teacher delighted in pronouncing my first name with a cod-French roll of the 'R', which really annoyed me) but I don't recall ever being bullied, not even on my very limited exposures to the sports field. I took A Levels in French, German, English, History and General Studies, which I passed, earning myself a place studying French and Italian at the University of London. It would appear that I was academically bright. I was invited to prepare for the Oxbridge entrance exams and I did for a while, but soon decided to not pursue this avenue: it was too 'elitist' for me. So off I went, to London University's Royal Holloway College in Egham, Surrey, and while it wasn't quite the bright lights I'd expected, it was a damn sight closer to them than Accrington could ever be.

I never really went back. And the reason for that, aside from the fact that I made my life in London, was that when I was at university my father died suddenly. I was doing my obligatory year of study abroad (in Paris) and I'd come home for Christmas. I was due to return to Paris to celebrate New Year's Eve there, so my father drove me to Manchester Airport. As we parted he gave me a big hug, which was a shock as he wasn't tactile in any way. Two days later he suffered a massive heart attack and died. Among his possessions we found painkillers and a little bottle of whiskey, so he was obviously fighting the pain – and typically in silence. After the funeral I returned to Paris and then to London and decided that my life would be there, not in Accrington.

There is a perception that if you're gay and you leave a small town for a big city, your life is somehow magically transformed into the paradisiacal existence you always wanted, but never dared hope for. Not true! And certainly not in my case. In my late teens and early twenties I knew I was different but I still hadn't quite worked out what that difference was. When I was at university there were a number of girls who expressed an interest in being more than just friends, but friends we stayed. And if I had thoughts about boys I lacked the courage to do anything about them, and for a long time too.

Why? Perhaps I was timid. Perhaps I didn't want to upset any-one by 'coming out'. Maybe – and this is a strong possibility – it was because I'd never been at all interested in the gay scene. I don't drink – I never have – and I don't go to gay clubs and bars. I certainly don't condemn anyone who does; it's just never been my thing. I prefer a night at the theatre or a dinner with friends. So the whole 80s scene passed me by completely. Do I regret it? Not at all – regret is like anger, a waste of emotion. There isn't much point looking back.

And there are other factors, too. Much of the gay scene is based on appearance – you've got to be young, slim, sexy, beautiful, and a stud. If you don't fit into that you risk being ostracised and I didn't want to involve myself in a so-called 'community' where that might happen. Sadly, it's also often the case with HIV. Gay men who are negative sometimes see gay men who are HIV positive as giving the community a bad name. 'You got yourself into that situation because of your risky behaviour, even though you knew the risks, and therefore it's your fault.' But more of this later…

I graduated in 1981. On the day of my graduation ceremony at the Royal Albert Hall, there was a general transport strike in London. The ceremony was followed by a service of thanksgiving at Westminster Cathedral. Mum, Philip and I made our way down the streets behind Kensington Gore trying, like the hundreds of other graduates and their families, to find a free taxi. Suddenly I spied a black cab with his light on speeding towards us. Still wearing my graduation gown I stepped into the road and waved my arms to flag him down. As he drew up I leant in his window and asked "Can you get us as quickly as possible to Westminster Cathedral?" Smiling, he replied "Any friend of Batman's is a friend of mine, get in!"

I graduated at a time of a major economic recession in the UK. Nobody wanted to employ a modern languages graduate and so I had a succession of temporary jobs: bank messenger in the City and then filing clerk for the same bank (where I was told to file all the correspondence under the initial letter of the sender, mostly other banks. I took it upon myself to file the Bank of America under 'A', the Bank of Canada under 'C', and the Bank of Ireland under 'I' and so on and was sternly rebuked for not having filed them all under 'T' for 'the'…) I was a tour escort for coach tours across Europe for mostly middle-aged Americans getting their first taste of the continent – 'twelve countries in seventeen nights'! I wasn't particularly good. I managed to leave people on top of mountains in Switzerland, on sinking vaporettos in Venice, and being beaten up by transvestite hookers in Paris. I had carefully done my research and written out little index cards to remind me of the highlights we were passing through. But sitting at the front of the coach I would fall asleep and the cards would end up in a pile on the floor. Someone would shout out "Where are we now, Roland, what's that castle on the left?" I would scoop up a card, any card, and reply with confidence, "We are now in Silesia and that is the castle of Prince Heimlich, the Grand Governor, built in 1824." Cameras would click and notes taken. A few miles later we would pass a sign saying (in the appropriate language) 'You are now entering Silesia. Take the second exit for Prince Heimlich's castle' and some bright spark would point out with gusto that I had just told them that was what they had already seen. I would reply, "That was Upper Silesia. We are now in Lower Silesia, which was governed by Prince Heimlich's son, Prince Heimlich II." Again cameras would click and notes would be taken. I feel I may be responsible for a whole generation of American tourists showing their holiday pics to their families and sharing completely erroneous information. I didn't last long at that job…

During that time I became a Freeman of the City of Chester. A distant ancestor of my father had, back in the seventeenth century, been a whitesmith (now known as silversmiths) in the City at a time when the reigning monarch paid a visit. He made a set of ornamental keys to hand to the monarch and as a result was made a Freeman of the City and given the family name of Chesters. That honour has been passed down through the male line of the family. Philip was sworn in by dad at Chester High Court, but when my turn came dad was no longer around. Mum had to stand up in the Court and swear fidelity to the commonalty of Chester; not an easy thing to say for one whose native language is not English! I believe the Freemanship entitles me to carry a loaded firearm within the city walls of Chester and to drive my flock of sheep through the City Gates. As I possess neither a firearm (either loaded or unloaded) nor a flock of sheep I have yet to put this to the test.

My first permanent job was at Bentalls department store in Kingston upon Thames. They had decided to follow the likes of their more well-known competitors (Harrods, Selfridges etc) and recruit graduate trainees. Myself and one other were the first cohort. My colleague left after a few months. Bentalls only recruited one more year of graduate trainees and then dropped the scheme. I would like to think that it didn't have anything to do with me.

A variety of jobs followed until finally I found something that suited me. I joined the Institute of Linguists as an Exams Manager, just after they had launched a brand new suite of exciting language exams. A great deal of time, energy and academic thought had gone into developing these very cutting-edge exams, but relatively little time, energy and thought had gone into developing the systems to support the delivery of the exams. Question papers asking candidates to follow a coloured route on a map, but printed in black and white, do not instil great confidence in exam candidates. I was brought in to help resolve some of those issues. And there I stayed for the next twelve years, rising to the dizzying heights of Director of Examinations, and Deputy CEO. It was a time I greatly enjoyed, but it was a small pond and I wanted to swim in a bigger pond. So I left, to join the Foreign and Commonwealth Office (FCO) as a Language and Testing Specialist.

After a number of years working hard and enjoying the company of friends, I realised that I would, after all, like someone to share my life with. Finding this person would also involve my coming out to my mother, which I did. Like many parents, her overriding concern was not my sexuality as such. My personal happiness was what she was concerned about, and whether I might end up a lonely, sad, bitter old individual. I just wanted to say, "I have this boyfriend" and for that statement to be OK. No more, no less.

I met Graham, the first of my two long-term relationships,

through a small advert in *Time Out*. I replied to his advert and when we met we clicked straight away. He was awkward for a number of reasons, not least because a couple of years before we met he'd been in a bad car accident and had had extensive surgery, including restructuring of his jaw. He had a number of visible scars and had also lost his teeth in this accident, necessitating a full set of dentures. Such physical 'imperfections', for want of a better word, were immaterial to me. He was a working class guy with ambitions and he was exciting and fun to be with. He lived in Bromley, Kent, but didn't want us to live together as a couple so I rented a flat nearby and we ran our lives that way.

Our relationship had its difficulties, many of which were centred round Graham's anxieties over his sexuality. He found it incredibly difficult to discuss the subject with his family, and whenever we saw them I was always introduced as his 'friend'. If he ever had work colleagues round I'd either have to leave or hide in the bedroom until they'd gone. At the time, I didn't know any different and assumed that was the way it had to be. I didn't want to upset his family by stirring up things I had no control over. And I wasn't 'out' at work; that only came much later, when I joined the FCO. So we were both living in the shadows at a time when being openly gay was becoming more acceptable, but the stigma and fear around HIV and AIDS was tempering such openness with a great deal of hatred, suspicion and misinformation.

After five years together, such pressures, and Graham's concerns about his sexuality, led to the inevitable and we broke up. It was a sad end to what had been a good relationship, but perhaps I should have been more surprised than I was when he rang to say that he'd introduced his aunt (his mother had died by this time) to his new… girlfriend. What can you say, other than 'happy for you…'? And I was, almost. But we never spoke again.

The end of the relationship was also the end of my time in Bromley. Other than Graham I had no reason to be there, so I left the flat and moved in with my mother, who had moved to Surbiton after the death of my father. I wondered if I would meet anyone else but I didn't go looking, undoubtedly because I felt I'd been burned once and was unwilling to repeat the experience.

Then one sunny day in the summer of 1996 I decided to take a walk along the Thames in Surbiton, on a path called Queen's Promenade. Perhaps I should have known… I'd taken a book and when I reached a bench with a pleasant view of the river I sat and began to read. Minutes later I saw a man walking toward me in the direction of Kingston. He was a tall, handsome broad-shouldered guy and as he passed our eyes met. We smiled…and that was it! We chatted and realised that although we lived just streets away from each other we'd never seen each other before.

I noticed straight away that Richard had a lovely accent. It was Barbadian, he told me. He'd been born and brought up in Barbados, had moved to England as a young man and never returned, aside from visits to his family. We both liked travelling, theatre, amateur dramatics and music, though our tastes around the latter were wildly different, as we would later discover. Before long we were a couple, Richard's charm and sincerity easily winning over my mother, who also fell in love with him I think!

Like me, Richard wasn't one for the 'scene' and at last I'd found someone I was completely in tune with. Eventually I moved into Richard's ground floor flat and when it became available we purchased the flat above it and combined the two, giving ourselves a very comfortable living space. We travelled, we enjoyed eating out, seeing shows and meeting up with friends. In short, we were happy – blissfully so. Until…

CHAPTER THREE

What do you do when you're told you have a life-changing illness like HIV? Run around, scream and shout and tell the world that it's so unfair? Or don sackcloth and ashes and join a silent order, forever in penance for your wickedness?

Everyone is different, and if you're reading this as a HIV positive person and you think, 'Oh yes, I did that!' then good on you. As they say, it's not what happens to you in life but how you look at it that counts and if yelling to the gods was your approach, so be it.

My own reaction is probably rather underwhelming (at least in the context of what is meant to be a dramatic story). I just went to bed and slept. I was so ill and so tired that anything else would have been a waste of energy. Maybe I just didn't care anymore and in some small way I was relieved that, finally, someone had told me for definite what was wrong with me, and that I wasn't going mad.

For the purposes of this book I contacted again the consultant who had suggested that I should take the HIV test, and sent him the chapter detailing the diagnosis, just to check that my recollection of the events is accurate. He replied to my email as follows: "I have had the chance now to read the chapter and also go through your medical notes from the time. It is so well written. Emotive, very realistic. I don't really have anything to add as you've described it so well.

Reading your email gives me enormous pride in my job as a doctor. I would prefer if you took out my name from the book. It is really an issue of confidentiality and all my patients need to know that I will be 100% confidential in dealing with them." I have to respect those wishes, of course. But I shall always have enormous gratitude towards him for, quite literally, saving my life.

I remember that first weekend as a mixture of relief and fear. 'I'm going to die in two weeks,' I thought. 'Well how about that?' Most inconvenient, and most regrettable too. How could I have been so stupid? How – HOW!? – did I manage to get HIV? I'd never slept around and neither, as far as I knew, had Graham or Richard. But here I was, a man in his forties with a stable partnership, a decent job, a pleasant home life – what on earth was I doing with HIV? The whole thing was unfathomable.

And I felt guilt. A whole heap of guilt for the way Richard had taken on the task of telling me. Somehow, he'd persuaded the specialist – against all medical protocol – to give him the diagnosis so that he could tell me. And I felt terrible he was ever put in that position. That, truthfully, is my biggest regret of the lot. The man I love having to tell his partner that he faced – at best – an uncertain future…well, I don't think I could have done that. And kudos to him that not only did he tell me with love and understanding, he also managed to not to look like he had the weight of the world on his broad shoulders while my mother and brother were having their coffee in our living room, unaware (as was I at that point) how dramatically life was about to change.

I was desperately worried for Richard. At that time, he hadn't been tested for HIV and he hadn't seemed unwell…but of course, you can have HIV without feeling unwell. The thought that I might have infected him was mind-blowingly horrifying. Fortunately, he never lost his cool for a moment and focused all his attention on me. Again, the greatest love and respect to him for being so measured while in the eye of the storm.

Quickly, the practicalities kicked in. I wanted to be cremated, not buried. I didn't want a religious ceremony. Oh and no flowers: such a waste. But what would we tell people? In a way, I didn't care so much about it at that stage. If I died soon, at least people would know that I wasn't a hypochondriac after all. The tiredness, the under-performance at work, the dizzy spells, the head pains, the confusion; I sometimes wondered whether everyone thought I was just making all this up for attention. Well, now they wouldn't. But did I really want my epitaph to be 'poor old Roland Chesters – he died of AIDS, you know'?

Ah, the 'A' word. At the beginning, no one even mentioned it. Officially, I was seriously ill with a HIV-related condition. The big 'A' wasn't breathed of, at least not in my presence. To talk medically for a moment, the HIV virus attacks CD4 cells, which are white blood cells that protect your body from infection. When you have a CD4 count (a test that measures the number of CD4 cells in a sample of your blood) the results you get determine your body's ability to tackle the infection. So the higher number of CD4 cells you have, the more able you are to fight infections, including HIV. The average CD4 count for a fit, healthy person is usually around 1000. According to the British HIV Association (BHIVA) HIV becomes AIDS when your CD4 cell count drops below a certain level and at the time I was diagnosed, in September 2006, the treatment guidelines recommended that medication should start when the CD4 count dropped below 300. The AIDS definition was when the cell count dropped below 200 and below 100, the chances were that the infected person would not recover. At the moment of diagnosis, my CD4 count was a mere sixty-two.

So yes, I did have AIDS, of that there is no doubt. Much later on my journey I asked my specialist about it and she replied in the affirmative. "Yes," she said, "it was AIDS and you were lucky to survive. But we don't tell people that."

The debate around labels such as AIDS will come later in this book. For the moment, it's enough to say that I was very, very poorly with an infection that was threatening to kill me at any moment. An appointment had been made for me the following Monday at the Wolverton Sexual Health Centre within the nearby Kingston Hospital and, shaken, stirred and everything else, I just about managed to attend with Richard in tow. It was a two-storey building and I was so weak I hardly knew how I made it up the stairs. Actually, I do know –Richard hauled me up. I simply couldn't walk.

The Wolverton Centre was housed in a somewhat dilapidated building on the extreme outskirts of the hospital, squashed in between the carparks and the smokers' shelter. I'm not sure if it was deliberately placed so far out of sight of the rest of the hospital in order to ensure that those affected with some kind of sexual health condition did not mingle with the rest of the general hospital clientele, or whether to spare the blushes of those having to access the centre. In either case that aim was not met as, when I attended, the smokers' hut was regularly filled with those desperate for their nicotine fix who, I am convinced, spent their time speculating on the reason for each person's visit to the 'clap clinic'. Since those halcyon days the Clinic has moved into a brand new facility in Kingston Hospital. But still…built on the extreme edge of the hospital, equally isolated, but now far removed from the smokers' hut.

And yet, despite my extremely dire state of health, this is where my recovery began. I was assigned to Dean Thomson, a specialist HIV community nurse, who would administer my drug treatment and generally be my guiding light. "We're not going to let you die," he said when we first met. I probably cried at that, and whenever I think about it now I have the same reaction. And he was as good as his word. Richard later told me that he asked to see Dean privately, separately from me, so that he could get a clearer idea of what the real prognosis was. I admire his courage.

In a later chapter Dean will describe his method of working, and his approach to me as his patient, but suffice it to say that for many months ahead he was my knight in shining leathers. On a near-daily basis he turned up on his motorbike at our home with my cocktail of medication. The neighbours must have wondered…

But I'm getting ahead of myself. Before the drugs were dispensed it had to be determined which would be appropriate for my condition and if any of those would cause an adverse reaction. Luckily, the ones I was prescribed would not cause such a reaction, so in a deep well of darkness that was something, at least. At first I was on a cocktail of Combivir (an antiretroviral) Kaletra, Septrin Forte, Loperamide, Domperidone (which sounds like Dom Perignon, but is far less fun) and various multi-vitamins. Naturally, there would be side effects including nausea, dizziness, lethargy, etc, but as I'd been having all those anyway anything else didn't seem to matter.

I was diagnosed with HIV-related encephalitis. A rather nasty infection that in my case attacked cells at the base of the brain, causing it to swell. Side effects include confusion, disorientation, fits, weakness, personality changes, memory loss, disruption to the motor skills and difficulty speaking. Ah! That would be me down to a tee then! Before the diagnosis I didn't really think to Google such symptoms but had I done so I might have had an inkling of what was the matter with me, which is more than any specialist had that I'd seen. Don't get me wrong, I'm not bitter about it – much – but an earlier diagnosis, even of encephalitis alone, would have triggered immediate treatment and I wouldn't have been at death's door before anything was done.

Anyway, now we knew what it was all about, something could finally be done. The drugs were prescribed and the most immediate treatment was a lumbar puncture, which would determine how far the infection had spread because there was a concern that I may not walk again. Nice... The cheery young South African chap who carried out the lumbar puncture looked at my notes and said, "Oh! I see you're on HAART."

Well, I didn't quite understand what he was saying and I thought that 'heart' might be an Afrikaner expression for 'happy'. "Yes, yes!" I smiled back, thinking that positivity was the answer in this situation. Little did I know that in this context, 'HAART' stood for Highly Active AntiRetroviral Treatment. He must have thought I was nuts. Perhaps I was, and if you thought about the implications of a lumbar puncture long enough you'd go nuts. You absolutely cannot move a muscle when the needle is inside you because if you do, it can connect with certain nerves and, in extreme cases, paralyse you. Altogether, it's a pretty unpleasant experience but after I'd had it I learned that the infection hadn't gone so far down the spine that it was irretrievable. So it was a grim procedure, albeit highly necessary.

Having been tested for any potential resistance to the medication, I started taking the antiretroviral tablets on the Wednesday or Thursday of that week. There was no discussion around this; it was a case of 'get the hell on with it'. These days, there would be a conversation on this subject, depending on how far the disease has progressed, because once you start taking such drugs you can't stop. That's you for life, unless you want to see your CD4 count drop accordingly. So I took around thirty tablets three times a day and felt absolutely, shockingly awful. The side effects were very unpleasant indeed, and dealing with a regime of so many tablets to be taken at highly regulated times was very difficult, particularly in my state of health. To make matters easier Richard sorted out the pills into a docket I'd been given by the hospital. Just working out how to open and close the caps on the little plastic trays was difficult enough for me. I had never been able to easily swallow tablets. As a child my mother had resorted to every means imaginable to get me to do this – crushing or pulverising them, hiding them in food I liked, dipping them in honey, but to no avail; I would gag and refuse to swallow. But now I had no choice. Swallow – or die. Quite simple, really. The tablets have to be taken at the same time every day, or you start to develop resistance to them. Remembering the times (remembering anything, really) was an issue for me, so Richard bought me a wristwatch with multiple alarms. I still have the watch. I don't need to use it any longer, taking the tablets at a set time has become second nature, but some things, some memories, are too valuable to be disposed of. Some tablets had to be taken before food or you would throw up. It did amuse me that one of the drugs that was made by a French pharmaceutical company suggested in the accompanying literature (literally, a small book) that it would suffice to eat a 'croissant' to ensure that nausea did not occur. Yeah, right because everybody has a café just round the corner with an endless supply of fresh croissants!

Bless him, Richard became my de facto carer. Life was going to get so complicated and yet he rose to the occasion wonderfully. Anything fresh I ate from now on had to be washed in boiled water so Richard went out and bought a huge pan, and brought it home with a big ribbon tied around it. The house needed to be totally germ-free and sanitized, and so Richard donned the Marigolds and got to work. I was capable of absolutely nothing, not even showering, and Richard had to help me with even the simplest of such tasks. How he coped so patiently I don't know and in the midst of all this he himself had to be tested for HIV. Fortunately he was negative, but goodness knows what was going through his mind.

It was important that I ate healthily and so Richard turned his not inconsiderable culinary skills to creating tasty nutritious dishes to tempt me to eat. I had lost a great deal of weight and had little appetite, but he persevered. Oddly, I seem to recollect that many of the dishes were of a blueish-green hue. He had been advised to add spirulina powder to my diet. Spirulina is a natural superfood that would add to my healing process. I did, however, draw the line at eating blueish-green porridge.

The days passed in a kind of haze. There were occasional moments of clarity when I had the strength to think, 'Well, what now?' Mostly, though, I felt completely flattened both in body and mind. I barely had the energy to ponder the next few hours ahead, never mind the rest of my life. And yet, 'life' was what I was still experiencing. Despite the gloomy outlook, I wasn't dead and as the days turned into weeks and the drugs got a grip of what remained of my immune system, I discovered that I wasn't ready for choosing the post-funeral sandwiches quite yet.

Was this a surprise to me? Yes, possibly. I was hoping for the best, but preparing for the worst, which I think is a common experience among people diagnosed with all forms of life-threatening or life-changing conditions. At the beginning I fully expected to die, but as time went on a glimmer of something more optimistic began to manifest itself. I was holding on by my fingernails, yet realizing that I also had a bit of a toehold, albeit one that seemed intangible. That doesn't mean to say I was at the stage where I was thinking positively or trying to visualise a glass half-full, or whatever. At this stage, my own personal glass was all but empty. Whatever future I had looked bleak; I would be on treatment for the rest of my life, and whatever quality of life I might have looked to be in very short supply. I had Richard, of course, but I even had doubts about that. "Please don't kick me out," I pleaded, that first weekend after the diagnosis.

"Don't be ridiculous," he said. "Why on earth should I kick you out!? We're together, aren't we? So we'll see this through – together."

I wasn't so sure. I needed him more than I needed anyone, but felt I'd let him down badly, horribly. Previous to my diagnosis Richard and I had, as I've mentioned, volunteered for the Food Chain, a London-based organization which at the time provided a hot Sunday lunch to people living with HIV and AIDS, and living in isolation at home. We were delivering the food, and during our rounds we'd quite often hear stories of relationships going wrong following diagnosis as the reality of the situation kicked in. Many of our customers were single, with no partner (or anyone else, seemingly) to care for them. Would I be in this situation too? The thought turned my stomach.

Yet he made no judgement about me and throughout his period of unemployment looked after me as though it was his full-time job. He kept a detailed record of the results of all the tests I had taken, and another meticulous record of all the medications I had to take. Around a month after diagnosis we were told by the clinic that I could start to venture out of the house. In my new state it was important to acclimatise to the world around me and as I didn't want to end up a recluse. So one weekend Richard decided we would drive up to Nottingham and stay in an anonymous chain hotel. On the Friday morning I woke up with the most enormous rash, right across my chest. I was convinced it was skin cancer, and completely panicked, thinking this really was the end. We rushed to the clinic and, after an examination by the lead doctor, was told it was shingles, nothing more.

"You're not going to die," she said, somewhat unimpressed by my hysterical reaction, "and really you should have seen the GP instead." Today, that's exactly what I would do but at the time I thought the slightest thing was a death sentence.

Not that shingles is a picnic, of course. We went to Nottingham, but because the rash is highly contagious we had to put a blanket down the middle of the bed so we didn't touch each other. I had a rotten few nights' sleep, which turned into weeks of poor sleep, which turned into years of the same. In the decade since I was diagnosed I can count on fewer fingers than I have on one hand the number of nights that I've slept through. I'm usually awake around 3am and quite often don't go back to sleep until the following night. I'll have weeks and weeks of this, then suddenly I will crash. Hey ho…

And so the day trips continued. Richard would wrap me in a blanket, pop me in the car and drive us to the seaside where we'd sit like a little old couple, just watching the waves. Simple pleasures, but wonderful too. I can remember some of these excursions. Some I cannot. I still have memory blanks. Richard will say, "Do you remember we did this, met those people, went there?" and try as I might, I can't. It's slightly scary to have lost entire episodes of one's life. Disappointing too! Some of those sounded like good times – shame I just can't remember. It's only when Richard reminds of the couple of thousand pounds that he said he lent me that I begin to smell a small rat…

But the going was tough. To paraphrase some other erstwhile author, 'It was the best of times, it was the worst of times'. Absorbed in our struggle to come to terms with what was happening, our relationship grew stronger. United against a common enemy, isolated from the realities of a 'normal' life, focused on achieving small steps, and celebrating each small step as a major accomplishment brought us closer together. I wanted to do something to show my appreciation for Richard, but I couldn't go out on my own. So I ordered an extraordinarily large bunch of flowers to be delivered to the house. In that bunch were three branches of twisted bamboo. The flowers faded and died, but the bamboo branches flourished and are still going strong. Life continues…

And yet I was overwhelmed with huge tidal waves of despair. The long trail of mornings I woke at 3am and padded downstairs to sit on the sofa and cry, alone in the dark, huge gut-wrenching sobs. I was in a place I never imagined I would be in. A place I definitely did not want to be in. The sense of loss of control. The confusion. The bleakness of it. The re-evaluation of what life is – or is not. The grieving for what I would probably never have now. The paradigm shift in terms of my expectations that had been so suddenly thrust upon me. I was bereft. If I did live, would I be able to work again? What would I be able, or not able, to do? If I couldn't work, how would we survive? I could not see any happy ending to this. And always, always, the never-ending questioning cycle of 'Why? Why me? What have I done to deserve this?' This was undoubtedly the darkest time of my life. And nothing can change that. Ever.

I was scared of somehow infecting Richard too. I wasn't as well informed then as I am now about how HIV can be transmitted. I knew the essentials though, like many other people. During that autumn our garden fence blew down. I was never particularly skilled in the dark arts of DIY but I struggled out into the garden to give Richard moral support in putting the fence back up. I manfully insisted that I could hammer a few nails into the fence but in so doing managed to bang one of my fingers. My yelp of pain brought Richard running, but the blow had also drawn blood. And I panicked, yelling at Richard to not come any closer, to stay away so that the (relatively small amount of) blood would not go anywhere near him. He told me to stick my finger under the cold tap in the kitchen and then to wrap it in a paper towel. The bleeding was quickly staunched and I felt somewhat foolish and determined to better educate and inform myself.

In December of 2006 Richard's brother-in-law died of cancer in Barbados. It was not unexpected and we had discussed what he would do when the inevitable happened. Of course he had to go back to his family, taking his mother (who had come to stay with us for Christmas) with him. I could not go – I wasn't allowed to fly. They left on Christmas Day. I had taken a taxi on Christmas Eve with my mother to go and pick up some Christmas gifts for Richard and he opened them quickly late that evening. My brother drove Richard, his mother, my mother, and me to the airport to wave them off early on Christmas Day, and after they'd gone I came back to the empty house and just wept. It was Christmas – my first, post-diagnosis – Richard, the only person who knew the full nature of my illness, was away, my mother and brother didn't know my status and I felt utterly, completely isolated. For the first time since diagnosis I really was alone. Up until then Richard was there, or Dean, or other medical staff.

And, to make things more complicated, we were having the wooden floor upstairs replaced and the builders were due on 2 January, before Richard's return. He had managed to move all the furniture before he left, but there was an eight-foot, fully decorated Christmas tree to contend with which he didn't quite get round to.

"Sorry," he said, "you'll have to sort that thing out."

Well, I was having problems just getting myself up and downstairs, never mind hauling anything else around. So I phoned Richard to tell him.

"There's no way I can move it," I said, "I can barely stand up. I'll just have to delay the builders' arrival, that's all."

"You can't do that!" Richard replied. "They've given us a slot! It'll be months before they'll be back again. You'll HAVE to do something with it."

The conversation ended. Richard has a great love of After Eight Mints and as a Xmas stocking filler I had bought him some, but obviously he had not had time to eat them before the rapid departure to Barbados. I do not care much for them. But on that occasion I decided to eat some of them and ended up scoffing the lot – and feeling rather sick. However, fuelled by an excess of chocolate mints, I looked at the tree. 'Yes, I will do something about it,' I thought, and promptly pulled it over. It crashed to the floor, damaging the lights and the decorations. I gathered up those and dumped them in the upstairs shower. Then I phoned Richard to tell him that I'd sorted it, and that the builders could now arrive on time. And that I had also eaten all his chocolates. He was pleased that the tree was down and slightly less pleased that all his chocolates had disappeared. But he was not so happy when he arrived home to witness the mess. Which goes to prove that even in the most catastrophic of health-related situations, normal domestic issues still have a habit of continuing!

CHAPTER FOUR

For many people, the letters HIV invoke the three big Victorian taboos which linger long after that era has passed, namely sex, homosexuality and death. No matter how 'HIV friendly' we've become as a result of efforts by organizations and individuals (rest in peace Princess Diana, you did a lot for us) the subject still isn't much talked about in 'nice' society, and those of us who need to disclose our status still feel a huge amount of stigma when faced with this very real challenge.

In later chapters we'll talk about the practicalities of this so for now I'll relate my own experiences of disclosure. First though, a word about the diagnosis itself and the question that is not often spoken by sensitive people, and indeed does not need to be asked but is often at the back of their minds – 'Exactly HOW did you get HIV?' In the last chapter I mentioned that at the beginning I had no idea how, when or where I'd contracted it. All I knew was that I was furious about it. My despair and anger were almost overwhelming; there were times that I'd get up at 3am and just cry and cry. I felt that I'd stolen my own future, that I'd ruined my life. At those times I was bereft; in other moments I was furiously angry, to the point where I'd break things around the house because doing so gave me some kind of relief. Eventually Richard took to putting sticky notes on various nick-knacks, saying things like 'Please don't break this, Aunty Maud gave it us,' or 'You can break this because it came from the pound shop'. So I'd break it (or not) then go into the garden and scream and shout. The neighbours must have thought I'd completely lost it. I was raging, but against what? Against the world and against me for being so stupid to get into this situation?

After Richard was tested, with a negative result, I was relieved that I hadn't infected him. We were officially, and to use the correct terminology, a 'serodiscordant couple', but I prefer the much more user-friendly term, 'magnetic couple', i.e. one positive and one negative. But also I was still apprehensive that this might be the point where our relationship could fracture. 'Who wants to care for at worse a dying man and at best, one whose future is very uncertain?' I thought. Well, the answer was that Richard did, and thank goodness for that. But there was still the question of where I'd contracted HIV. The severity of the diagnosis put the source of the infection way back before the ten years Richard and I had been together. Graham and I had been together for five years and it had been our first relationship for both of us. I assumed at first that it was sexual, and that it must be connected with Graham. We had had unprotected sex, and I cursed myself for being so stupid. But then I began to look at the situation more closely. As I've mentioned, two years before I met him Graham was in a terrible car accident which required extensive surgery and blood transfusions. While we were together he developed night sweats for no explicable reason, to the point where I encouraged him to see a doctor. Graham was told that this was as a result of the extensive anaesthetic used in the operations but looking back, I can now see that night sweats are a classic symptom of HIV. And so, if he hadn't cheated on me (which I presume he hadn't, as he was so uncomfortable about his sexuality) I can only assume that he caught HIV via a transfusion, in the days when blood wasn't screened properly for the virus. Over the years I have tried to track him down, without success. I'd like to think that doesn't mean he's no longer around, but I just don't know.

Does any of this matter? No, of course not. Did it make me feel any better, assuming my own infection had come via a transfusion? No, it didn't, because I was in no position to be making moral judgements about 'good' or 'bad' ways of being infected, and there is still no justification for such judgements. Who cares how you got it, it's what you do next that counts. And no matter that there was an element of 'bad luck' rather than abandoned irresponsibility within my diagnosis, I was still spittingly angry. Angry with Graham, angry at myself, angry at all the medical people who'd missed what now seemed to be the blindingly obvious symptoms of an HIV-related illness. 'Ice-pick syndrome' indeed...I felt like planting an ice pick right at the heart of the medical establishment for being so stunningly stupid. And this anger took a long, long time to dissipate. Years in fact, and not before I'd also been diagnosed with Post-Traumatic Stress Disorder (PTSD) resulting from the HIV diagnosis.

So there were lots of bitter pills to swallow, medical and metaphorical. And sooner or later I had to tell people, who might ask (or at least wonder privately) "Oh Roland how DID you get HIV?"

I decided to go for a soft approach. I was already signed off at work with viral encephalitis (i.e. the brain's functions were impaired by an infection) so I needn't go into too much detail with them for the moment. Sexual health records are kept separately to any other medical records and are always highly confidential, so work would not have been told the full diagnosis by the medical professionals caring for me. Having said that, if anyone at the FCO had cared to investigate the stamp on the doctor's sign-off statement, which shouted 'THE WOLVERTON CENTRE' in large letters, they may have wondered why I was being treated for a brain infection at a sexual health clinic. Luckily, no one did, and I was able to get away with the minimal amount of information for the time being.

When Richard went away to Barbados that first Christmas I had plenty of time to think about disclosure and whom I should (or should not) tell. I didn't want to tell my mother, as she was aged and infirm, and I didn't particularly want to tell my brother for the moment, as I wasn't sure how he'd react. I felt terribly alone and lonely, despite the presence of my mother and brother. I missed Richard terribly. On New Year's Day I went out for lunch with Simon, a friend of Richard and mine. Like others, he was well aware that I had been seriously unwell, and like others he had only been told of the encephalitis. Over that meal I revealed the truth of my diagnosis to him. He was curious, concerned, sympathetic and understanding. A first hurdle overcome. However, I did want someone close to Richard to know, in case the worst happened and he needed immediate support. So I decided to tell Maddy and Suzanne, a lesbian couple who are Richard's oldest friends in the UK and a few months later, as I was helping them to make preparations for their civil partnership ceremony, I told them. Or rather, I told Maddy. She told Suzanne in the car on the way home. I got a phone call shortly after they left the house from Suzanne, in tears, telling me that they still loved me. And they have been constantly incredibly supportive and caring since then. I'd done this without Richard's knowledge but once done, I 'fessed up.

"OK," he said, "I understand why you've done it, but I want you to tell your oldest friends just in case anything ever happens to me and you need support."

Typical Richard, always thinking about someone else! So I agreed and contacted my oldest friends, Pip and David. As well as being close to them I'm godfather to their three children, all now in their twenties. When I was asked to be godparent to their first-born

I knew I was gay but it was pre-Graham and I wasn't exactly out and proud. So when they asked me I said "yes...but a) I'm not religious and b) I'm gay."

"Fine," they replied, "neither is an issue."

And so I became godfather to them all and had many happy times in their company, watching them grow up. Eventually they all met Richard and were very happy for us both. I told Pip and David about my HIV status but at that time we agreed we wouldn't tell the children. As they got older, and I was open about my status and was posting updates on Facebook, I suggested that 'now is the time.' Their parents agreed, and so we met in a cafe and I told them one at a time. And of course, they were fine. A bit surprised, a bit shocked, but they took it all in their stride. 'What the heck,' was the reaction, 'let's just get on with it.'

Back in 2006/2007, telling people wasn't quite so easy, nor did I expect such a matter-of-fact reaction. I was off work for four months and, if I'm honest, didn't feel much like going back. True, the medication had taken a hold and I could walk and talk (and I still wasn't dead) but the psychological fallout of the diagnosis was all-enveloping. There were days when just lifting my head from the sofa was enough; the idea of catching a train, walking into a big Government department in Whitehall and managing people was laughable, had I had the energy to laugh.

Richard, however, was having none of it. Aided and abetted by Dean, my community nurse, he persuaded me subtly and not-so-subtly that going back to work would be good for me. I wasn't going to sit around moping forever, he insisted, and I needed to start looking outwards. So, in early January 2007, four months after diagnosis, I did as I was told and went back to the FCO, initially working two days a week (mainly from home, it must be said) for four weeks of a phased 'return to work' programme. After this I would increase my hours to four days a week, working from the office for four hours at a time. Richard too had found himself employment and was back at work.

Before I returned to work I felt it necessary to disclose my status to my line manager, Marta. She was also a friend and had, up to this point, understood that I had encephalitis only. When I told her the truth she was shocked, but also concerned and empathetic. However, she felt she had a duty to inform Human Resources, which I didn't disagree with. They knew I was gay: under their rules I had had to disclose this to them in case I was 'compromised' in any way placing myself open to blackmail and therefore a potential threat to national security. This may sound draconian until I tell you that until 1991, being gay debarred you from working there at all. I guess they still hadn't forgotten the days of Guy Burgess et al...

So she did tell HR, and at the same time she also advised me not to tell the people I managed because she wasn't sure 'how they would react.' She wondered if they might not want to use the same cup as me, or share my keyboard. Or indeed, shun me altogether.

Now, I should have thought this through objectively, telling myself that it was almost 2007 and the great falling icebergs and tumbling tombstones of the first AIDS awareness campaigns in the mid-1980s were long behind us. We knew, didn't we, that HIV didn't jump from cup to cup, chair to chair or keyboard to fingers? By now, we were a bit better than that; more clued up, less 'ignorant' than the politicians of the 1980s would have us believe. Weren't we?

However, at the time I was feeling terrible; quite depressed about everything and uncertain as to whether I'd even make it into work, never mind do my job and manage other people. So in my naivety I agreed that my colleagues shouldn't be told about my status. Mistake Number One.

Mistake Number Two happened when I was asked by work to

book an appointment with an occupational health therapist who had been contracted externally. She had some background in HIV work she told me, albeit twenty years previously when treatment was in its infancy and the prospects for HIV/AIDS patients were nowhere near as good as they were in 2006. During our first conversation, which consisted of a barrage of questions from her, most of which I could not answer, she referred to my notes and let me know that I had something called Progressive Multifocal Leukoencephalopathy (PML). I had no knowledge of this, and told her.

"Well, according to your notes it's what you've been diagnosed with," she said.

This was news to me. I thought I had viral encephalitis. That's what I'd been told. What was PML? I went home and did what we'd all do – and probably shouldn't – and turned to Google for help. What I read turned my bowels to water.

> Progressive multifocal leukoencephalopathy (PML) is a rare and usually fatal viral disease characterised by progressive damage (-pathy) or inflammation of the white matter (leuko-) of the brain (-encephalo-) at multiple locations (multifocal)…
> In general, PML has a survival rate of 10–20 percent in the first few months and those who survive can be left with varying degrees of neurological disabilities.

So, far from getting better, I was probably going to deteriorate. In a state of complete meltdown I phoned Richard who, at that moment, was just about to choose a sandwich from Tesco for his lunch.

"I'm going to die!" I sobbed. "The OH doctor told me I've got something called PML and I've Googled it and the survival rate is rubbish. What are we going to do!?"

Richard, of course, was his usual calm, collected self. "I'm just going to pay for this sandwich,' he said, "then I'll ring Dean and find out what's going on. How does that sound?"

Richard to the rescue, again. He phoned Dean, who was apoplectic that this person had spilled the beans to me. Even so, I hadn't been told by the HIV specialist and I was annoyed about that. I guess now that PML is another way of saying that I had AIDS and, as I've mentioned, when I asked my specialist the question much later on she admitted that this was the case. They just don't like to tell you that, as it's a little bit frightening. And it's just another label, another pin to add to my lapel: gay, HIV positive, living with AIDS, battling PML... Soon I would be running out of lapel space. And the occupational health therapist also offered me another lapel pin to add to my collection: she diagnosed me with PTSD (Post- Traumatic Stress Disorder) – the ordeal of my diagnosis had taken a toll. She explained that this could partly explain why I was getting up at 3am: I felt that I needed to complete things, get things done and draw a line under them because I didn't know if I would have any more time to be able to finish stuff. Helpful explanation, but it didn't stop me still getting up in the small hours most days.

And so 2007 got underway and, as planned, I made a gradual return to work. To say it wasn't easy is an understatement. In my world, everything had changed. I could never be the same Roland Chesters who took an HIV test some months back, not suspecting for a moment that it would be positive. My colleagues were pleased to see me back and, to them I hadn't changed. To all external appearances, I looked exactly the same. They knew I had had encephalitis, but nothing more. And like all staff do when the boss returns, they would be coming to me with petty issues and minor squabbles in the hope I could resolve them. None of this was their fault; it's what goes on in workplaces all over the world. But I felt like shouting, "Oh, just get over it! Life's too short!" I couldn't do that, though, as

I'd been advised not to. If I'd done so, I believe the situation would have been much different.

The medication was still giving me awful side effects, including pain, fatigue, sickness, lack of concentration, memory impairment and so forth. Not ideal for someone who was meant to be managing others, and there was no way I could return full-time for a while. A different OH doctor had also told the FCO that I should cut back on my hours, with more emphasis on working at home, thus avoiding the stress of commuting and managing other people. I proposed that I could carry on my specialist examinations role without having to manage others but my employers, perhaps understandably, were concerned by the situation.

After seven months of a reduced return to work programme I received an email from a senior manager who pointed out that under the terms of the return to work programme I should have been back to full-time hours within 12 weeks of a return to work date. Then she added this:

> Officers are normally expected to receive pro-rata pay for the hours they are able to work if they are unable to increase to full-time within 12 weeks. Even allowing for some flexibility which is afforded to those officers whose medical conditions are deemed as being likely to be covered by the Disability Discrimination Act, it would appear you have exceeded the reasonable amount of time which is permitted for rehabilitation purposes and at full-time pay.

And with that, this manager ordered that I take another medical to 'seek a view as to when you are likely to be well enough to work full-time.'

The message was clear: get back to work full-time, or else.

I hadn't been told about the twelve-week rule and to be informed four months after the event was appalling. I said this and as a consequence they backtracked a little, telling me I'd receive full pay until after the examination. And so began months of examinations, assessments and questionnaires that would determine whether I was fit to return to work in a full-time capacity. Don't get me wrong; this is what I wanted. I didn't want to be an invalid, lying around all day feeling sorry for myself. I'd always worked hard and I saw no reason not to now. I just wanted my employer to understand that my life was different now, and that some adjustment should be made for that fact.

It was upsetting and stressful and worrying. But oddly enough, it didn't hit me anywhere near as hard as a letter I received on Friday 20 July 2007. A letter which, despite (perhaps because of) its plain English and matter-of-factness, seemed to destroy whatever hope I had left for my future.

CHAPTER FIVE

In its entirety, the letter from Dr Allison Beardall, my HIV consultant at the Wolverton Centre said this:

16 July 2007
To whom it may concern
    This is to confirm that Roland Chesters is a known HIV positive patient at the Wolverton Centre, Kingston Hospital.

Yours faithfully,
Dr A Beardall

The reason for the letter was a quite legitimate one. I was desperate to get as much information as I could gather about HIV and AIDS and I'd signed up for a Terrence Higgins Trust course for newly diagnosed people. Although I wasn't 'newly' diagnosed in the strict sense, I'd had enough of reading half-truths and downright misinformation on the web and wanted some answers from people truly in the know. However, I needed a letter from my clinic to confirm my HIV status before the course would accept me. And, on this unseasonably wet Friday morning in July, here it was.

It was the first time I'd seen my HIV status in writing. I'd seen references to encephalitis, and I knew what medication I had to take and when appointments had been made, but up until now I'd never seen the words 'HIV positive' in stark black and white associated with my name. I felt I had been handed a death sentence. 'This is what is going to kill me,' I thought. 'I survived those first few months and I can walk and talk but eventually, inevitably, this is what will finish me off.' And it would undoubtedly be long and slow, painful and degrading. I didn't want that.

A month previously we'd celebrated our civil partnership at the Lovekyn Chapel, a beautiful medieval building, the venue of the first grammar school in England, given that status by Elizabeth I. We'd been planning this for a while, and during the period Richard was away in Barbados I'd done some research into venues and found this place. It was ideal for our needs so I booked it and, despite everything else, we planned for a very happy day. My aunt and her partner and my cousins were coming over from Paris for the event, as was Richard's sister from Barbados. I did keep asking Richard if he was sure he wanted to go ahead, did he really want to commit to someone whose future was, at best, uncertain? But in his usual way, he just said, "Oh, let's get on with it!" And so we did. The fact that the Registrar called Richard 'Richmond' twice during the ceremony, which could potentially mean that I am civil partnered to a town and not to a man, is immaterial.

At this point my mother, who was now eighty, was developing dementia and was quite unwell. However, she was in good enough health to attend, along with my brother, and she appeared to have a great time. I'm not sure she really understood what was going on, but she was all smiles and that is what counted on the day. Whether she'd have been the same had she known my status…well, she never did, because I didn't tell her. She knew I was unwell, but not to the extent that I had HIV. I felt there was absolutely no point worrying her, particularly at her age and in her condition. I saw a lot of her, as she lived just around the corner, and I simply didn't want her to fret. She had her own health to worry about, never mind mine. There were days when she would appear at the front door and bang to be let in, but I was too unwell, too engrossed in tackling my own demons to be able to face hers as well, and I would watch from an upstairs window as she walked unsteadily down the road back to her own home. I felt bad – I still feel bad – but I didn't know what else I could do.

Richard was at work the day I received Dr Beardall's letter and when he arrived home I acted as normally as I could. We had a straightforward sort of evening, ate dinner and went to bed. As usual, I was awake at around 3am so I went downstairs. After all the rain we'd had that summer, dawn was breaking on a warm, clear day, the first in ages. The world felt new, washed clean. And I thought, 'Why wait?' Hope had died for me that night, and without hope there is no future. I felt my life was broken and I didn't know how to stick it all back together. The appeal of oblivion was all too strong.

I dressed and let myself out of the house as quietly as I could, turning left at the garden gate in the direction of the river Thames. It was along the riverbank that I'd first met Richard, and it would be here that I'd bring our wonderful partnership to a close. I didn't want to put him through a lifetime of me becoming progressively poorly, unable to do anything or go anywhere. In short, I didn't want to be a burden.

I sat for a while by the riverbank, gazing into the water flowing by. The Thames looked so calm and peaceful, a fitting place to end one's life. I paused, then removed my pair of Timberland boat shoes. 'Too nice to waste in the water,' I thought. 'Someone else could enjoy them.'

I made to stand up, but as I did I heard a small noise behind me.

I turned, and saw Richard sitting a few yards away, just watching, and almost sensing what I was about to do. He got up, sat just behind me and put his arms round me.

"You know," he said slowly, "I can understand why you feel this way. But if you go ahead and jump into the river it's going to hurt me really badly. And I'll be so, so sad that you've gone."

"I just can't face things any more," I said. "I've got this thing that's going to kill me. Why hang around?"

"You don't know that it's going to kill you," he replied. "Not for sure. It could be something else. And even if it does kill you, it doesn't necessarily mean you'll die painfully or degradingly."

I looked at my shoes, forlorn on the bank. I didn't really want anyone else to have them.

"You know, Roland," Richard said, "whatever happens in the future, I just want you to be around. Come on, let's go home."

Like a child, I did as I was told. On went the Timberlands and we walked home, slowly hand in hand and in silence. In the days, weeks, months and years ahead there were still moments when I thought, 'What's the point?' but over time the thought went as quickly as it came. There is always a point, right up until the moment when there really is no point – and if and when that moment is reached then I will do something about it, as opposed to lingering in pain and suffering.

So that was a very low moment indeed for me, at a time when everything felt in flux. I went to work on the Monday morning and it was all, 'How was your weekend, Roland?'

"Well, I tried to kill myself, how was yours?"

I didn't say that, of course. I pretended that nothing had happened. I was pretending anyway, so another white lie wouldn't hurt.

Before I leave this subject, a word about Allison Beardall. Her letter might have caused me a sudden wobble by the banks of the Thames (which, I must stress, was no fault of hers – it was my reaction to it) but in fact she is one of my saviours. When I was first taken under the wing of the Wolverton Centre at Kingston Hospital Alli was on medical leave, so I only met her perhaps a couple of months after my diagnosis.

Tall, with long blonde hair and a calm demeanour, Alli sat with my extremes of depression, stress and sickness, listening to my questions and responding without hesitation, but with reassurance and positivity. One of the big differences I found was that Alli always gave the impression that she had all the time in the world to listen to all my concerns, hopes, fears. Unlike the four minutes you get with a GP, I would sometimes spend up to an hour with her. I would go prepared with a list of things to ask, report or comment on. They could be HIV-related…or sometimes not. And they would be dealt with, one by one.

The regular visits to the Wolverton would follow a pattern of being seen by the Clinical Nurse for the usual form filling ('have you taken all your meds?', 'have you missed any doses?', 'any change to your smoking/drinking/recreational drugs habits?'), weight taking and blood pressure monitoring. Then I'd be passed on to Alli for the discussion and reporting on test results from the previous session. Then on to the dietician for a lecture on 'good' eating habits, maybe a whizz past the clinic's psychologist to check on my mental well-being, before finding my way back to the clinical nurse for the bloods to be taken and finally, into the pharmacist on the way home to pick up the boxes and boxes of meds. The blood taking could be… difficult. I have 'rolling' veins. At the sight of a needle they roll out of the way! There could sometimes be as many as a dozen of those little bottles to fill and the only way to find an accommodating vein would quite often be to locate one in the back of a hand – and that's painful.

Over the course of time the only thing that changed was that the medication would be delivered to my home by a private service. The hospital encouraged this as it was less costly to them. The service provider would contact me to arrange a convenient time for delivery. I would be given a password to give to the delivery man. A plain white van would draw up outside the house and the plain brown wrapped box would be handed over to me on disclosure of the required password. I would then spend the next thirty minutes removing all evidence from the packaging that this was medication to treat HIV/AIDS, just in case.

I felt I could discuss anything (within reason!) with Alli. She remained a voice of sanity in my world that had somehow become, in some kind of way, quite insane. She always appeared to be as pleased to see me, as I was pleased to see her. When she decided to move from Kingston Hospital to Roehampton Hospital I felt that I had to follow her, even though Roehampton was more difficult for me to access. As sexual health records are kept entirely confidential to the particular clinic, my records could not go with either me or Alli from Kingston to Roehampton, so we had to reconstruct them together.

Eventually, the difficulties in accessing Roehampton when I was back to work became too much and I sadly discussed with Alli moving on to another HIV clinic closer to my workplace. Sexual health clinics are the only ones where it is possible to self-register and change as often as one wishes. Although, obviously, your historical records do not travel with you. Alli wrote me a letter of introduction to another HIV specialist she recommended at St Thomas' Hospital, ten minutes from my work at the Foreign & Commonwealth Office, and that is where I still receive my treatment.

Shortly after I left her care Alli decided that she and her family would relocate to the USA, given the changes that were – and still are – taking place in the NHS. What the US has gained from the decision, is, I believe, a great loss to the UK. I shall be forever immeasurably grateful to Alli for the time, patience and care she showed to me. And I am sure I am not alone in saying that.

After that attempt to, quite literally, drown my sorrows, I decided that I could not live my life afraid of what might happen. And so I did attend the Newly Diagnosed course, along with twenty or so other people. Apprehensive, nervous, bewildered, timid, shy and somewhat overwhelmed would describe all of us, I guess. And yet, at the same time, somehow liberated. Coming from a place where I felt so alone, so isolated, adrift in an ocean of my own personal experiences that nobody else could possibly have any idea of what they were, to finding myself surrounded by others who were also afloat in that same ocean was so empowering. With the best will in the world, nobody, NOBODY, however supportive, however empathetic, however caring, could possibly even touch the sides of the depths of emotion that I had experienced. But these people had. We shared a common vocabulary. We came from the same place. We had found a safe haven with each other. And over the next six weeks we were able to share fears and concerns, causes for celebration or trepidation and develop a new sense of identity. An identity that includes HIV but is not dominated by it. A person 'living with', not 'suffering from'. An identity that is in control of our destiny. That has a future. Whatever that may be. An identity that has hope as its middle name.

And for me that started an ambition. Seeing the impact that this course had had on me and my fellow delegates I decided that I too wanted to be in a position to enable that to happen to others. I spoke with the course facilitators about how they had been recruited to be in that position. They said, and I agreed, that it was too early in my HIV journey for me to consider taking on that role, but to come back again in a few years' time. I made a note in my diary. And I did go back. And in so doing I have been so lucky to be able to empower others to make that step forward into their future with confidence, head erect, looking others straight in the eye, saying 'this is who I am'.

Terrence Higgins Trust also ran, at that time, a similar course for the negative partners of newly diagnosed people. I suggested to Richard that he might find it useful to attend as he would find information, resources and support there which I was not capable of providing. He attended the first session of the course and decided that it wasn't for him.

I also applied to receive some counselling from one of THT's trained counsellors, specializing in providing that service to HIV positive people. In order to access the service you had to have an assessment interview. I remember very clearly being asked by the assessor the status of my relationship with Richard. At one point he directly asked me if I loved Richard. It was the first time anybody had so bluntly asked me that question. And I prevaricated. I clearly recollect having a Celia Johnson moment from *Brief Encounter* and giving an appropriately middle class response to the question: "I'm terribly, terribly fond of him." Fortunately the assessor pursued the question and eventually got me to clearly state "Yes, I love him." And I'm proud to be able to say that.

So life went on, in the usual whirlwind of work-related examinations and assessments. Health-wise, I was still all over the place; the occasional days seemed to pass without incident, but the majority of the time was spent feeling nauseous and dizzy, and in a state of blurred vision and fatigue. Travelling into work was so, so difficult and yet I was doing my best to be as 'normal' as possible under the circumstances, perhaps not quite grasping at this stage that 'normal' was a thing of the past. An FCO external assessment of my condition in late July 2007 recommended that I could work two days a week at home, and two in the office, with an increase to five days (three at home and two in London) within a month. The doctor told senior managers that I should avoid coming into the city during rush hour (stressful enough for the healthy, as half a million daily commuters will attest to) and that having flexibility to work at home would assist a return to full-time work. And still very few people really knew what was up with me; a situation I was finding increasingly difficult to cope with. 'Better they knew and understood,' I thought, 'than leave them wondering and speculating...'

I had to go into hospital for a couple of weeks for tests to try to work out why I had a 'shaking leg'. My right leg would jiggle uncontrollably. It was exhausting and uncomfortable and the doctors couldn't work out why, and how to stop it. So Alli referred me to St George's Hospital for assessments. On arrival at the hospital I had to complete a form which asked for, among other things, my GP's contact details, which I duly supplied. The tests were done and proved inconclusive (the tremor disappeared of its own accord a few months later) and I thought nothing of it until one evening a few weeks later on a packed commuter train home I received a call on my mobile from my GP. He was also the GP for my mother and my brother and I had not informed him of my HIV diagnosis or of the encephalopathy because all of my health-related issues were being handled by Alli. I also didn't want my HIV status to go on my NHS records as that would impact on such things as insurance. I answered the phone and the Doctor told me that he had received copies of test reports from St George's, which said that I was HIV positive and was this true? Pushed against the sweaty armpits of my fellow commuters I felt I had no choice but to enlighten him. He was immensely supportive and said that this information would not appear in my NHS records, for which I was grateful (and also the reason why I cannot give his name here). Over the years, as I have become more open about my status I have no problem with the GP knowing. The surgery I attend has a number of GPs so you never see the same one and each time I do have to go and I am prescribed some medication I have to remind them to check for contra-indications with my HIV medication.

Not all those in the medical profession are so forward thinking. Before my diagnosis I had been seeing the same dentist for many years, being treated for, amongst other things, gum disease (very common amongst HIV positive people). A few months after my diagnosis I returned to continue my treatment. She started off by asking the routine questions about medication and I gave her the names of the new medicines I was now taking. She disappeared into a back room and after a few moments sidled back in clutching a copy of a medical encyclopaedia. "You do realise" she whispered to me (why she was whispering I have no idea; we were the only two in the room) "that these are medications for HIV?". For one brief fleeting moment I was sorely tempted to deliver an Oscar-winning demonstration of horror, shock and grief, rolling prostrate on the floor. However, common sense prevailed and I revealed that I was indeed aware of that fact. "That being the case", she continued' "I'm not able to treat you now. You will need to return at the end of surgery so that we can be sure the practice is appropriately sanitised before the next day." I was shocked and left there hearing my leper's bell clanging in my ear 'unclean, unclean'. I did return at the end of surgery – but only to inform her that I would no longer be a patient of hers; if she had no confidence in her clinical procedures then how could I be confident of not catching something from any of her other customers with a highly infectious conditions of which she was not aware? Sadly, I was to learn that this is not an uncommon experience for HIV positive dental patients.

Just over two months after our civil partnership ceremony I met again the same Registrar who had officiated at that event, but this time to register my mother's death. Whilst I was very sad indeed, I was also glad that she'd seen Richard and I go through our civil partnership, and even more pleased that she'd always accepted who I was, and had loved the person I'd chosen to spend my life with as much as I did. Mother had been in a home for ten days to provide us with some respite care. On the morning of the day she died I had gone for a swim, as it was a day I was not working and swimming was part of the regime I had been advised to follow to get some return to health. Whilst swimming I was struck by the thought that I had to go and see mum in the home immediately. The feeling was so strong that I left the pool, dressed and caught the bus to her home, stopping briefly en route to buy her some of her favourite flowers: red carnations. On arrival at the home I was told she was in her room because she was not feeling well. She was dozing, propped up in her bed but woke when I entered her room. She told me she was in pain, back pain, but had been given painkillers. I held her hand and told her how important she was to me. She drifted off back to sleep and seeing her sleeping peacefully I left and caught the bus home. I had barely turned the key in the lock before the home phoned to say that mother had been found unconscious and taken as an emergency to Kingston Hospital. By the time I got there she was no longer with us. A heart aneurism. I got the impression that she had had enough, and simply turned her face to the wall. We arranged for her to have a humanist funeral. She probably wouldn't have recognised the term but she was, in many ways a humanist. The crematorium was packed out and we played Edith Piaf's *Non, Je Ne Regrette Rien*, which seemed so entirely appropriate.

Shortly after her funeral my brother and I had a sit down and agreed that we'd let out her property. However, it needed some repair and renovation work to bring it up to rental standards and as this might not be insubstantial Philip proposed that we arrange a joint mortgage to cover the cost. The major part of the cost was £36,000 to extend the lease.

Sensible enough, but there was a catch. To get a mortgage you need life insurance, and I couldn't get life insurance because…well, at that stage my life wasn't very insurable. And so I had to tell my brother. He was distraught.

Readers might wonder why I hadn't told him before. Weren't we close? Did I think he might let the secret slip to our mother? Or was it something else? My brother is a very sensitive person and I didn't want to hurt him, then or now. But there was no other way to tell him why I wasn't eligible for a mortgage and I did hurt him. He was enraged; very angry, very hurt and very disappointed in me. I think his anger came from somewhere deep; a place deeper than I can understand, and I think he felt he'd been completely deceived. I explained to him that I didn't think I could tell him because of his close relationship with our mother and there was no point in telling her because she had dementia and even if she'd understood all it would do would make her worry and what's the point of that? I said it had been my decision and that I took full responsibility for it. Richard also rang him in an attempt to smooth things over, but he was obviously still angry and we knew that we'd just have to wait in the hope that he would eventually understand.

A week or so later Philip sent me a message, asking to meet me for a drink in a local pub. I agreed, with an understandable degree of apprehension. When I arrived he offered his hand and I took it.

"How's the disability?" he said.

"OK," I replied. "I've not been very well at all, but…you know. It could be worse. Much worse, to be honest."

And so, from that day on, things got better between us. The

'thing' had been spoken of, Philip hadn't wanted to know the details but he had wanted to know how I was. And I was fine with that. Even now, when he rings up or calls, he always asks, 'How's the disability?' That's his way, and that's OK with me. I say 'I'm fine, thanks' and I am. I can't see the point of changing my response because it would only worry him if I became ill.

I discussed the writing of this book and the contents of this chapter with Philip. I wanted to make sure that he was OK with it. Sadly, this appeared to open old, unhealed wounds and Philip became very upset again. He asked me to include these sentences. 'As we didn't get a mortgage this left Philip in great difficulty to find the £36,000 to pay for the lease extension that we had signed off for and in the end he had to increase the mortgage on his own flat to pay for it. In the event as he did not have enough to pay off this mortgage increase he had to cash in one of his pensions, which left him in severe financial difficulties.'

He then later sent me an email which he titled 'Crying all afternoon', the contents of which are just too painful to share here. A few weeks after sending that email Philip had a major heart attack. His heart stopped beating for thirteen minutes and although he survived the attack, the lack of blood flow to the brain caused substantial brain damage. He was in intensive care for ten days and eventually transferred to a neuro rehabilitation centre. Philip had a second, fatal heart attack on 9 September 2018. I never had the opportunity to discuss any further the impact of my diagnosis on him. This shreds my heart.

Back to the summer of 2007. The medication I was on for encephalopathy and HIV was giving me horrible side effects, and when it was swapped that situation became even worse and I was trying to manage four people on a part-time basis while feeling totally chewed up and spat out. I made it clear to the FCO that

I was no longer able to manage people. It was a situation that was only going one way, and in the late summer a very strong 'suggestion' was put to me that it would be better for all concerned if I were to seek early retirement on medical grounds. Indeed, I was handed an application form that had been partially completed on my behalf.

I was still only forty-eight. Retirement felt like a thing that grateful elderly people did at the end of a long working life. I'd had seventeen years of specialist work in the languages field, work that I had enjoyed and been good at. Now, I was being told that I was no longer of any use in the working world. That my use-by date had well and truly expired. So here I was, completing the form, and feeling like I'd been handed a loaded revolver. But given how unwell I still felt, I couldn't see any other options. It seemed to be the easy way out and reluctantly, I took it.

In the form I explained that my condition wasn't completely stabilised and no one knew when I'd make a good enough recovery to come back to work full-time. I acknowledged that although I enjoyed my work, it had been made clear to me that a non-managerial role could not be created for me, nor could part-time, flexi-time or job-sharing arrangements. I concluded the form by saying that it was written 'with a heavy heart' and I prepared to pack my belongings to leave my place of employment forever.

CHAPTER SIX

The response eventually came back that my application for medical retirement had been accepted, although the committee noted that I did not appear to be overwhelmed with enthusiasm by the idea and suggested that all potential avenues had not yet been explored. It was accompanied by the calculation showing how much of a pay out I would receive. It was a pittance though hardly surprising given my relatively short tenure as a civil servant. Both of these stiffened my resolve to not leave, to not give up the battle, to stay and regain a degree of control over what I was doing, and restore some of my dignity.

Although I'd elected to stay with the FCO (perhaps *because* I'd elected to stay with them) they were sticking to their argument that my pay grade should come with managerial responsibilities that I ought to be carrying out. I understood this, but was still in no position to manage anyone. At best, I was just about managing myself. And still the people I worked with, barring more senior management, had no idea that I had HIV.

Truth be told, I didn't want to manage people. My managerial difficulties – and the fact they didn't know what was really going on with me – put my staff under a fair bit of pressure. I was hoping one of them might step up and take over my role, which would allow me to reduce my hours and my salary accordingly, but without being downgraded. I also asked about job sharing but because my role was a specialist one, apparently that wasn't possible. So none of these things came to fruition.

There was discussion after discussion after discussion. I joined Prospect, the trade union for professionals in the public and private sectors, and although they told me they didn't usually take on pre-existing cases they seemed happy to fight my corner. The union rep came along to various contentious meetings I had with HR. There were appraisals that appeared to attack me personally with little understanding of what I was going through.

Then there was a letter from the HR department which confirmed that I should be 'working standard hours' and that coverage of my managerial responsibilities when I wasn't working was potentially risking the health of my line manager. Well hello! My health was stressing me out too! This letter also advised me to bid for other jobs in the FCO, which was news to me. As a specialist in the FCO you did the job you were brought in to do until you left. Other 'generalist' staff changed jobs usually after every two to three years.

In the meantime, I'd started to get a little bit more active with my HIV status. Instead of sitting around moping and perhaps as a way of alleviating the pressures of work, I began to explore avenues that might help others in my situation. I did some training with the Terrence Higgins Trust to run a 'Positive Living Programme' for newly diagnosed people, and undertook an 'Expert Patient' training programme to help those having medical treatment for HIV/AIDS. I was also getting counselling from Terrence Higgins Trust and slowly learning to realise that regret and anger are two strong emotions that in themselves are pretty useless, but their strength can be put to positive use. I joined the FCO's LGBT support group and the Disability Advisory group, and I also went on the committee of the users' group (as in 'service user') at the Wolverton Centre in Kingston Hospital.

As a result, by early autumn 2008 I felt I was in a position to tell my work colleagues about my status. After two years, I was no longer on the return to work programme and I felt that it was right that they should know. My chance came at one of the Disability Advisory Group meetings, during which someone proposed a lunchtime briefing session for any staff member interested in invisible disabilities, mainly around mental health. A couple of charities were supplying speakers and colleagues were going to talk about their own personal experiences. I mentioned that I could tag on something about my personal experience of HIV and AIDS to the session and bring in some speakers. In effect, I was going to 'out' myself. But I didn't want the people I managed to find out about my full diagnosis from seeing the poster advertising the event. I had, though, created a small card that slips into my wallet (it's still there) which states that I am HIV positive and on medication, in case I am ever caught in an accident with spillage of blood.

Marta, my line manager and the person who'd advised me not to tell them, was concerned. She thought that by telling the whole truth I would be vulnerable to comments, actions and even thoughts and, as she explained, was just looking out for my well-being. I appreciated her concern but I was two years on from initial diagnosis and my thoughts had changed from, 'No one should know!' to 'Why shouldn't anyone know?' I'd been very ill indeed but I'd survived and I felt I had something to share from this experience. I had walked in enough shadows as a closeted gay man in my youth and I wasn't prepared to have to do that again as a HIV positive person for the rest of my life. Marta was still worried but she agreed and so we called a departmental lunchtime meeting.

In a nutshell, I said that I was taking part in the disability awareness event, 'and this is the reason why.' And – surprise, surprise

– no one walked out, vomited, beat me up or insulted me in any way. In fact, there were more than a few tears and hugs, and a general sense of 'right, so that explains quite a lot then'. Their reaction gave me all the encouragement I needed to take part in the briefing session. In the event, none of my colleagues felt able to talk about their mental health experiences. But I stood up in front of a crowded room of about 150 people, talked about my diagnosis and the impact it had had and said that the FCO was effectively trying to get rid of me because I had HIV. I was extremely nervous. This was the first time I had talked openly about my diagnosis to such a large number of people. And once that information is made public, there is no taking it back. My ripples were starting to spread wider. But in making this information public I felt that I had effectively shot right through the FCO's argument in trying to get rid of me.

Two things happened. The first was that I started to notice my health improving. By this time I had probably been through about four or five different regimes of medication, having to be moved on because of the disastrous side effects. The first meds I was on had to be taken just before going to bed as they completely unbalanced me, and Richard would have to guide me up the stairs. They also gave me horrendous nightmares. The second regime gave me jaundice: colleagues would stop me in the corridor to ask if I had been on holiday I was so yellow. I was taken off the third regime as it was discovered they could impact on the heart (and I am in the 'at risk' category: male, over forty, overweight, history of heart issues in the family). And so it went on. Each new regime brought the initial nausea, diarrhoea, headaches. But now the meds had finally stabilised and overall I felt more positive (so to speak) about my diagnosis and long-term prospects. What hadn't killed me had indeed made me stronger, and I wanted to make a contribution to society based on that. And to my career.

The other thing was that an office restructure had meant

a job change for me. I was told that my job in language training was going to be cut so I was effectively being made redundant from that job. To transfer from being a specialist into a mainstream FCO generalist job you usually have to go through an assessment process but as a reasonable adjustment around my disability I would not have to go through that process, I would be allowed to go for a job at lower grade and I would continue to be paid the higher-grade salary. To that I said, 'Fine, bring it on.' This position was easier to manage, in all senses of the word, and I began to get a sense that my job, my health and my life were finally back on some kind of course. I accepted the chairmanship of the FCO's Disability Action Group and tried to give this forum a better and more effective voice when representing its interests to the FCO management. And that empowered me enormously and gave me the courage to find the voice to be able to say 'I'm HIV positive, deal with it'.

I became the FCO's Diversity & Equality Policy Officer. The role's focus was to tackle bullying, harassment and discrimination not just in our London base but in FCO outposts across the world. This was a challenging role, not least because bullying, harassment and discrimination can take many forms, and what we in the West mean by such terms might not necessarily be applicable overseas. One of the ways I set out to tackle these issues was to train up a group of volunteers representing a variety of different posts across a global network to become first response officers. These were people to whom an individual could go if they'd been on the end of inappropriate behaviour and discuss whether their grievance was relevant or not.

Two thirds of FCO staff abroad are employed on a local basis and, as I've mentioned, in different cultures there is a different un-derstanding of what bullying and discrimination is. Some cultures are very passive and whatever the boss says is right; in some lan-guages there is simply no terminology for bullying, harassment or discrimination. People feel unhappy but don't know how to express it. We had one issue connected with a post in Africa, where locally employed staff felt they were not being acknowledged as individuals because British staff didn't say 'Good Morning' to them personally, using their name. As we know, a 'good morning' in a British office is a general grunt in the direction of colleagues, and everyone accepts that, but it took on very different connotations in Africa and British staff needed to be aware of that.

I remember dealing with an issue in which the spouse of a British office had been asked to create a handbook for newly arriving British FCO officers at that Embassy and she'd written that, in the local culture, people often said 'yes' when they actually meant 'no' because they wanted to be seen as willing and civil, but that could lead to frustrations when people said they'd do something they didn't really want to do. This went on the local intranet and local staff who saw it were rightly aggrieved. So, trying to instil a certain amount of common sense and discretion was a big part of the job. Travelling overseas to certain countries as an HIV positive person can be fraught with difficulty as there are about 17 countries in the world which will not allow such people to enter. I was obliged by work to go to one such country but permission to do so was only granted on the basis that the Embassy there would ensure that I was escorted out of the country as soon as my work there was completed. I always travel with a note explaining that I cannot be separated from my medication – although it doesn't say what the medication is for.

There was a home role too, as I've mentioned. One World AIDS Day I thought it would be a good idea to ask the Terrence Higgins Trust to come in and do a lunchtime briefing about the impact of HIV/AIDS across the world. I was organizing it not only as Diversity Officer, but also as a colleague living with HIV and I put posters up around the London offices advertising this event and my role in it as a colleague living with HIV.

A day or so later I was horrified to discover that some posters had been slashed or defaced. Some others had been taken away by my line manager, who obviously didn't want me to see what had happened to them. I was very hurt and angry and a little bit scared, especially about the slashing which is such a physical act. I couldn't understand why if some people were so concerned they didn't just get in contact with me and talk. After all, my number was on the poster.

I decided to write an article for the FCO's in-house magazine, describing the impact the slashing of the posters had, not just on me but on anyone who might feel in a vulnerable position, health-wise. And, true to Civil Service bureaucracy, I was asked by the magazine's editor to write a response as Diversity Officer to my own article! In the circumstances, it was rather absurd so I asked my line manager to write it instead.

There was a bit of an inquest into who might have nobbled the posters and the powers-that-be concluded that it was likely to have been builders or some other outside contractors. I wasn't convinced; anyone coming into the FCO from the outside has to pass a lot of security clearance and no one goes around unescorted. And anyway, why would you risk a potentially lucrative contracting job by scrawling all over some posters? It didn't add up, but in the event, I didn't bother to find out who was the real culprit.

The following year I decided I wasn't going to organise a briefing for World AIDS Day. Instead, I put a box of red AIDS ribbons on the table outside my office with a collecting box. Later that day, one of my colleagues said someone had taken the box, thrown all the ribbons on the floor and walked all over them. It seemed so silly and unnecessary. If people had issues I considered it to be their problem, but I was there to help resolve them and my door was always open. I didn't bite!

I was approached by the Terrence Higgins Trust to participate in their publication 21st Century HIV, to tell 'my story', which I was happy to do. I was asked if I wanted it published under my name, or under a pseudonym. I was surprised – it hadn't occurred to me that I wouldn't want to use my real name, although I do understand and appreciate why others might not feel the same. On the strength of that publication I approached the Business Disability Forum (then called the Employers' Forum on Disability), of which the FCO was a member, to ask to speak to them about HIV/AIDS. They knew relatively little and were happy to take up my offer of delivering some in-house workshops on the issue for their staff and also to do a couple of dial-in masterclasses on the topic for their members. I was billed as 'Roland Chesters from the FCO' which caused great consternation in the office, in case, heaven forbid, I was seen as being the FCO 'expert' on the topic and so I was quickly rebilled as just plain old Roland Chesters. The telephone workshop was successful. Later that year the FCO submitted to the Business Disability Forum's annual Disability Standard – a benchmarking exercise of how disability inclusive an organisation is. The FCO fared reasonably well in the exercise and I was amused (bemused?) to read in the evaluation report "We thought that Roland Chesters' participation in EFD's internal training and our telephone tutorial for our members on HIV was an excellent way to demonstrate your commitment to disability." Seems like some organizations like to have their cake and eat it too!

A few minor setbacks aside, as time went on my health and general wellbeing seemed to be improving. Before I was diagnosed Richard and I used to take our bikes out regularly along the Thames towpath, but my HIV status and the encephalopathy put paid to that. However, my strength returned sufficiently to venture out once again and we set off one sunny afternoon for a short jaunt. And I fell off; not once, but twice. The first time I was overtaken by a platoon of Lycra-clad males, causing me to wobble and crash. They looked at me with a mixture of pity and contempt as I lay sprawled on the ground. Later on, I wobbled and fell off by Hampton Court railway station and was first-aided by a couple of elderly ladies who rushed to the scene. This time, it was extremely painful, especially around the shoulder area, and I was sent off to Ashford Hospital to see a surgeon, who recommended an MRI scan.

I wasn't particularly worried by this. Before and since my HIV diagnosis I'd had had so many scans I felt I merited a 'scan loyalty card': with every five scans, you get another one free! And in a strange way found them rather relaxing. I've worn glasses from the age of five and generally only take them off for going to sleep. So, when I do take them off I tend to fall asleep almost immediately – a kind of Pavlovian response, I think. Stick me in a scanner, where you have to take off your glasses and I'm out like a light. Before you enter the chamber the nurse usually asks what kind of music you'd like to be played on the headphones, and I always say 'classical' and as I lay dreamily in the Ashford Hospital scanner the strains of Vivaldi's *Four Seasons* and Handel's *Fireworks* drifted through my subconscious. The third piece was the choral version of the 23rd Psalm – the one that contains the line 'Yea, though I walk through the valley of the shadow of death, I will fear no evil: for thou art with me; thy rod and thy staff they comfort me.' And I thought, 'Do they have a playlist they use for people they think are goners?'

When the scan results came back they showed that I had a fractured vertebra. They also revealed that I had osteoporosis and atrophied ventricles, both HIV-related. Nice. The neuro-surgeon was keen to operate as he felt it was the best way to relieve the on-going pain

I was experiencing in my arm but it would take several months on a waiting list. The pain was so dreadful that I elected to go on the waiting list. In the meantime, I had to wear a neck brace as any abrupt movement could impact on the fracture and cause me to become paralysed. I wore the brace for over six months. If anyone at work asked me what I'd done, I started off by replying it was a fracture caused by HIV-induced osteoporosis but I soon tired of seeing their eyes glazing over so I instead took to replying 'it's the hang-gliding, you know', which would usually elicit a degree of interest. Even so, this was no joke. The neuro-surgeon warned me that there was an outside chance of being almost totally paralysed as a result of the surgery and as the date for the operation loomed closer I had the distinct feeling that I'd be one of the small minority who drew the short straw and became paralysed. And I couldn't face the thought of that.

For the second time in my life, I began to consider ending it. I contacted Dignitas, the assisted-suicide organisation in Switzerland, and obtained the necessary paperwork. I gave this to Richard, along with the fee, and told him that's what I wanted should I become paralysed. His response was that we would deal with it as and when the worst happened. But I felt the need to be prepared in advance so, I asked a friend, who initially said she'd accompany me then a week before I was due to be operated on told me that she didn't feel able to do it. I appreciate her position; I doubt I too could do something like that for someone dear to me. By now I was seriously stressed and mentioned this to Alli Beardall, who suggested I get a second opinion and recommended someone she knew. I duly trotted along to this second neuro-surgeon who took off my neck brace and examined me. He said that I'd certainly had a fractured vertebra but that it was the neck brace that was leading to pain via a trapped nerve. "If you stop wearing the neck brace," he said, "you'll be fine." I did as I was told and he was right. I didn't need the operation and I didn't need Dignitas. And I took great delight in phoning the first neuro-surgeon to tell him the good news!

Unfortunately, my work-related difficulties continued with no apparent sight of resolution, despite thoroughly enjoying my role as Diversity & Equality Policy Officer. I was assigned a new line manager who was determined to make her mark as a decisive and brilliant operator and very quickly expressed concerns about the standard of my written work. One evening, as we were leaving for the day, she handed me a copy of the FCO's performance improvement process which, in a nutshell, said that unless I pulled my socks up I might lose my job.

I was very distressed because I'd always considered that I had a decent standard of English, both written and verbal, and that I was able to express myself in both. I also knew that in the lead up to the diagnosis of both HIV and HIV-related encephalopathy I'd suffered from poor concentration, some difficulties with speech and short-term memory loss. I spoke with the FCO's disability consultant and again, I had to see an external specialist, this time for a psychological assessment. I showed strengths in vocabulary, reading, spelling – but weaknesses with non-verbal reasoning and working memory. All of which, the assessor concluded, was consistent with a diagnosis of dyspraxia, gifted to me by the onset of encephalopathy. Thanks for that...

CHAPTER SEVEN

Dyspraxia is, according to the Dyspraxia Foundation, 'a form of developmental coordination disorder (DCD), a common disorder affecting fine and/or gross motor coordination in children and adults. It may also affect speech.' Although the exact cause of it is hard to pinpoint, it is thought to be a result of disruption in the way messages from the brain are transmitted to the body.

For me, it affects the way I absorb, retain and reproduce information, and I have coordination problems too – hence the 'falling off the bike' episode. However, because the FCO has a specific style of written communication, it was most noticeable in work, hence the opinion that I 'couldn't write properly'. As I've mentioned, it's most likely that the dyspraxia was brought on by encephalitis but thinking back, I was a very clumsy child. I was hopeless at sports and ball games and it's likely that I had a dyspraxic tendency then which was later exacerbated by the encephalitis.

Now I find it difficult to read and retain what I've read. Writing isn't easy either, and I constantly have to take notes and highlight and rewrite in my own words. Then there are the memory problems. I used to be keen on amateur dramatics but these days I'd be pushed to remember the second spear-carrier's lines! This goes hand-in-hand with facial recognition – I even struggle to remember who my neighbours are. Richard is very good; when we see someone I ought to know he says, "Now smile, that's so-and-so…" And I do, and all is well until Richard isn't there and I completely walk past the neighbour without acknowledging them, and they think I'm the rudest person in the street. It's tedious and boring, and sometimes I wonder whether it's really dyspraxia and encephalopathy or just creeping old age! That said, when I was first diagnosed with dyspraxia the FCO's disability consultant wrote to my HIV specialist asking whether it was caused by encephalopathy. The specialist replied in the affirmative, copying me in and adding that 'Roland will never be normal again.' My first reaction was, 'Great! Another label.' And then I thought, 'Who cares, and who wants to be normal? Normal is a setting on a washing machine! Normal is boring!' And now my mission in life is to never, ever, be normal.

But I understood why she wrote it because it was important for the FCO to understand that HIV-related encephalopathy had brought it on. This meant that reasonable adjustments had to be put in place to enable me to continue working in that department. Chiefly, this consisted of voice recognition software so that I could create reports etc without having to type. This was extremely useful, except that it had one disadvantage; the difficult line manager could hear everything I was saying, and when I wasn't using it she'd be on my case, asking me why it wasn't being used; the implication being that I was idling. I also couldn't use it to write any emails about her. That became very difficult and unpleasant but luckily my 'tour of duty' in that post came to an end and I got another job within the FCO as a learning and development advisor. Another two years went by in a job that suited me reasonably well with a very supportive line manager, and that I enjoyed. During that time I studied for and passed qualifications with the Chartered Institute of Personnel and Development (CIPD). My health was also improving (or stabilizing, at least) and after almost eight years of living with HIV I was at the point where I'd accepted it for what it was and had adjusted to the demands it made upon my life. There are occasional small blips such as when I developed Bell's Palsy: within an hour or so the left-hand side of my face became paralysed. Apparently it is pretty common to people living with HIV, but to me it was just another reminder of what potentially could still happen. The psoriasis comes and goes, the bone and muscle pains are controlled by regular free sessions at the British School of Osteopathy, the stomach issues trundle on, the fatigue is ever present and the high cholesterol levels are controlled by yet more tablets but…hey! I'm alive.

Then the FCO went through one of its regular phases of restructuring and they wanted back office people (like me) to go into front office jobs, for example working for policy desks and suchlike. That had no interest for me at all. At the same time the chance to take voluntary redundancy came up; incidentally this was on 1 September 2014, the eighth anniversary of my diagnosis. Each year it is a reminder of how far I have come – but also of how much is, or is not left. A time for remembrance and reflection.

I had a meeting with my line manager and said, "I think it's time for me to go, to do what I want to do." And put it this way, there wasn't a huge amount of resistance put up against my suggestion. We parted amicably and I'm sure they were as glad to see me go as I was to leave. I'm aware I made life difficult for them sometimes but I'm also proud of the fact that I left the place having made several important changes to the way the FCO works, including the one which now says that if a disabled person is in a job they are happy with and they are doing it well, they don't have to fulfil the FCO requirement that positions must be changed every few years. It makes sense for the individual: having to 'explain' your disability to a new set of colleagues, ensuring that reasonable adjustments (if they are needed) are put in place is exhausting. It also saves the FCO the costs of having to re-implement whatever adjustments are required in a new setting.

The offer of voluntary redundancy couldn't have come at a better time. For a while I'd been toying with the idea of leaving to set up a training and coaching consultancy business. I didn't want to be an employee again and wanted to capitalise on the work I'd done in the FCO, the voluntary work outside of 9–5 and the qualifications I'd gained during my working life. Naturally I wanted to work specifically around issues of diversity, inclusion and disability; my experiences with HIV and its impact upon my life and work more than qualified me to do that! However, as with all new businesses you take what you're offered and I was prepared to be flexible.

I called my company 'Luminate', with the intention of shedding light upon my clients' issues and making a positive (no pun intended) difference in their lives. At the time of writing, nearly three years into self-employment, I have worked for a variety of organizations including training consultancies, training foundations, charities, government departments and individual clients, delivering coaching, workshops and motivational speaking on a range of issues. Given that the work is about diversity it is often diverse; one day I may be delivering anger management skills to a group of adults with learning disabilities and the next I will be training corporate managers in understanding the implications of unconscious bias.

I still wake up early thinking that the diary's looking a little lean for next month, and I miss the comfort and security of a monthly salary, but there's nothing to beat the freedom and variety that my work now gives me. Being dyspraxic I need to plan very carefully and make sure I have everything in order, otherwise I will get on the wrong Tube line (!) so I have to think about it all carefully. It does do my head in at times, but in a good way I guess.

If I may talk about voluntary work a little, let me just say that to assist people in this way is incredibly rewarding and personally enriching. As I mentioned at the start of my account, Richard and I volunteered for the Food Chain, a London-based organization which provided a hot Sunday lunch to people living with HIV and AIDS. That was fine, but it was nothing compared to the experience of volunteering and assisting others who are in exactly the same position as you. Perhaps it was the shock of contracting HIV or an 'It's not going to beat me!' attitude that I had to adopt as a survival mechanism, but not too long after my diagnosis (and after I'd experienced it myself) I set up a group for newly diagnosed people at my local hospital. For me, it was vital to know as much about this illness as possible, because after all, knowledge is power, and to know what you're experiencing is to take back some control of that experience. Initially I started working with mixed groups, then later on with gay men only.

I discovered that Positively UK trains peer mentors who will attend HIV clinics and will approach people to ask them if they want any help or support. And those mentors would describe how hard it is to engage people. So I trained as a peer mentor and as part of that mentoring I put together a workshop for them all about emotional intelligence. And I used a snappy title: 'Knowing Me, Knowing You – Aha!' I've absolutely no idea where that came from (thanks, Benny and Bjorn...).

I then delivered newly diagnosed workshops, initially for THT, then for Positively UK who, instead of holding these over six weeks, like THT, they do it as a non-residential weekend. Later, I joined the National Long-Term Survivors Group (and was eventually asked to be Vice-Chair), where I also delivered residential newly diagnosed weekends. Although the core themes and the (hoped for) end results are pretty much the same between these organizations, the difference lies in the timescale of the delivery. I think the THT course works well because it gives time for people to go away and reflect, then come back the following week with insights or questions. It doesn't work so well in that sometimes people disappear, perhaps because they can't quite handle it or weren't altogether ready for such a course.

Residential courses are often more intense. You're away from home, perhaps in the middle of nowhere, and while you're free to go, the logistics of leaving can be more difficult. For forty-eight hours you're living and breathing your newly diagnosed status and so the emotional intensity is so much higher. That can be difficult for some, and liberating for others. It depends on the person you are. I do remember one young man coming on the course who, having embraced his status, posted it on Facebook over the course of the weekend for the whole world to see. He worked in a nursery school and, when parents found out, the school told him that they had no choice but to ask him to leave. Beware the ripples...

But at least he recognised his status and felt able to deal with it. Those who already feel isolated have a much harder time with this. I remember one chap coming on the THT course who'd been diagnosed some years previously and was obviously having difficulties coming to terms with it. One of the sessions was about safe sex and he absolutely and utterly refused to attend that session. He intimated that he'd not been infected through sex and because he worked in a hospital I assumed he might have caught it from a needle. Gently I asked him but he said 'no', it wasn't via a needle. He never disclosed how he was infected, which was fair enough, but his general sense of denial worried me a lot. Some of the guys on these courses are so very young. On one occasion one of the evenings of the workshop fell on the day of one delegate's twenty-first birthday. What a way to spend such an important occasion. He insisted that he would attend, so I bought a cake and candles and made sure that his birthday was celebrated, whilst at the same time feeling incredibly sad for him.

I met people from all walks of life on these courses. When I was facilitating a newly diagnosed group at Kingston a young woman came to one session and told how, having disclosed her status to her friends, she had been banned from her local pub and her children were being victimised at school. Her front door was sprayed with graffiti and she was shunned everywhere she went. Her partner had knowingly infected her and she wanted him prosecuted for that. I had to explain that while she could seek justice ('recklessly' infecting a person with HIV is a criminal offence in the UK), a defending barrister would pull apart her sexual history in open court. Unfortunately she didn't finish the course and I never found out what happened to her.

Extreme reactions from other, non-HIV positive people are, sadly, all part and parcel of this illness. THT used to run pop-up testing sites in shops and offices, trying to raise awareness of HIV by encouraging people to be tested. I volunteered to help out at one of these pop-up clinics in Dalston, London, and we would approach people walking past. You had to be kind of careful who you approached of course, but some people would be outraged by the mere fact they'd been approached. "How dare you?" they'd shout before stamping off. Others would say, "I don't need to be tested – God will save me." "Really?" I'd think, "I didn't know God was a condom…"

I am a member of the Positive Voices Panel for THT and often, when delivering a talk on HIV/AIDS to a group I start off by asking if any of them know of anybody living with HIV. They usually do not. "Would you be able to recognise if someone has HIV if you met them?" Some think yes, some think no, some don't know. "Well, now you have met someone living with HIV" and at that point you can hear a pin drop. Perhaps they expected to see someone who looked very unwell or someone who they would automatically know was infected. At a recent talk to a group of nursing students at a central

London college, one of them said that the only thing he wanted from the talk was to know for sure whether HIV really exists. To mark World AIDS Day (1 December, every year) I recently volunteered to act as one of the hosts for an exhibition of UK AIDS Memorial Quilt panels in Westminster Hall, the very seat of Parliament. The exhibition was not only to remember World AIDS Day, but in particular that day in 2017 as it marked the thirtieth anniversary since the UK government launched its public information knowledge campaign on HIV and AIDS; the now infamous 'tombstones and icebergs' adverts on TV and leaflets thrust through every letterbox in the land. Hence the reason why the authorities allowed the exhibition to take place in Westminster Hall. One of the quilts on exhibition particularly affected me. The quilt itself had been covered over by a rough sheet to which had been pinned this note: "This Panel was made by a Friend for a Friend. The Parents do not want this panel shown anywhere. The Stigma still exists. Until this changes this panel will remain covered. A Red Ribbon is not enough. The Quilt is not enough. What will it take? Attitudes must change." Further information on the Quilt can be found at http://www.aidsquiltuk.org/about/.

The work I do now with Luminate is not specifically for people living with HIV; it's for anyone with any kind of disability, and disability awareness raising within organisations. It's about trying to help people with disabilities realise what abilities they do have and getting employers to recognise that is the case. The coaching I do is about helping people to regain the confidence to approach an employer and help them to identify the skills and attributes they have which would be useful in the workplace.

I understand the challenges employers, particularly small-to-medium enterprises (SMEs) may have with disabled employees. Unlike larger organizations, which often have their own in-house HR teams to deal with issues of disability, SME employers have to personally make sure that the organization keeps going and can't afford for employees to work at less than full capacity. My role is to help their thinking around that by seeing what can be done in terms of reasonable adjustments i.e. working from home, flexible working and changing duties to some degree. That said, HR departments in bigger organizations need to be up to speed with ever-changing legislation around the rights of workers with disabilities, but also understand that a supportive culture needs to be created too. There is a difference between legislation and culture and while you might be compliant it doesn't mean you have a culture that is supportive of people with disabilities.

What else? Well, aside from my professional and volunteering roles I have also trained as a Humanist Celebrant for funerals. Odd, you might say, considering my brush with death. Wouldn't I rather be immersed in life? Well of course I would, and I am, but death is a fundamental part of life as is birth and it's important – vital even – that it is handled with the same understanding and sensitivity, and as a crucial rite of passage.

When my father died he had a traditional Anglican funeral service with a vicar who didn't know us as a family. During his address he got my father's name wrong – twice – and almost forty years later I still remember that lack of familiarity. My mother was raised a very strict Catholic and when she married my father she had to renounce her Catholicism so she could get married in an Anglican church. Her experiences as a Catholic marked her quite badly and in her later years she was very anti-religious. She wouldn't quite recognise the term 'humanist', but that's what she was so we had a humanist funeral for her and it fitted her to a T.

Even before I became ill I was sure that I didn't want the same reception from the church as my father had received. After my diagnosis this was brought into much sharper focus and following my recovery I decided to do the Celebrant training. I hope I have a certain amount of empathy and, again, my experiences with HIV and the gamut of emotions that can come with it have helped me, I think, to understand the needs of dying people and of those left behind. In my early twenties I was a Samaritan for five years, so I picked up essential listening skills from that experience.

Lately I've started to speak about my experiences in public and I hope I haven't bored anyone so far! People have been very encouraging and helpful with constructive feedback. At the time of writing it's still early days but I've enjoyed the experience and hopefully it's been useful to at least someone in the audience, so we will wait and see.

Recently I volunteered, along with another member of the National Long Term Survivors' Group, to rattle cans at a performance of *Rent*. This musical, set in a 1980's squat in New York and dealing with the impact of AIDS on a group of young people, was on for a short run in a small off-West End theatre. We had permission to do a collection at the end of the penultimate performance. The theatre asked one of us to go on stage at the end of the performance and say a few words about why we were collecting, and I agreed to do that. However, the performance started about an hour late. Five new understudies needed to be put through their paces. This meant that the show would finish very late and audience members would be anxious to escape to get their transport home. The storyline is very emotional (certainly when I saw it as an audience member I, along with many others, had tears in my eyes) and the cast got a standing ovation that night. I had a fully prepared little speech, but when I was thrust onto the stage all I could say was "Hello, I'm Roland and I'm living with HIV and AIDS" and the whole place just erupted. I was overcome but managed to stagger through some information about the group and why we were collecting. I rushed round to the exit to join my colleague with a collecting tin as the audience left.

Soon we were so inundated with people wanting to give us notes that we couldn't fit into the tins that someone fetched some (clean!) pint glasses from the bar which made it easier to collect the money. Many people said kind words as they left. One lady said to me "The play made my cry and then bugger me, you made me cry again." We collected nearly £400. I shall be forever grateful.

Forgive me if I've indulged in a little trumpet-blowing over the last few paragraphs. As I said in my introduction to this book, I don't feel I'm special or in any way 'unique'. Millions have been through what I've been through. Some have died; many have survived. I'm an ordinary person – even if I'm not quite 'normal'! But I do think it's important to emphasise that there IS life after a life-changing diagnosis of an illness such as HIV. Ironically, being HIV positive has had many positive points for me. It has given me a focus and it has given me a voice. It has exposed me to so many different people from diverse backgrounds that I might not otherwise have met. It's given me the drive to realise that I can make some contribution to society. It has taken me in a direction I would never have dreamed of going; it has led me down paths I never thought to tread. I wouldn't wish my condition on anybody but at the same time I'm not ashamed to be HIV positive. I'm not quite there with having pride in it, but I'm certainly not ashamed of it. If there is any pride involved, it is that I'm proud of what I've done with my diagnosis and what I hope to do with it in the future.

I count my blessings every day. Sure, there are still days where I feel exhausted – physically, emotionally, mentally. Days where I feel ill or in pain. Days when I can't help but think how relieved I will be when this is all over. But they are increasingly few. My health is stable, I have a wonderful and supportive life partner, a nice home, interesting work and good friends. I live in a country where treatment is freely available. I look forward to meeting more inspirational people that I can learn from. I also look forward to that dream world where everybody is recognised and valued for what they can contribute. Sadly the world isn't like that and you can't change human nature but that doesn't make me pessimistic. I still believe there are beacons of light out there, and I've met many people in this context, so if we all keeping beavering away, meeting people's basic needs and refining upwards we will all be in a better place.

I have a favourite saying: 'Life isn't about being afraid of the thunderstorms. It's about learning how to dance in the rain'. There have been quite a few thunderstorms in my life and each time I got out there and danced, each time learning new steps and a different rhythm. There will undoubtedly be more thunderstorms ahead. So if you see me out there, dancing in the rain, please come and join me. There is nothing worse than dancing alone.

The next part of this book broadens my experience to take in issues which will be familiar to those who have a life-changing condition, and those who care for and love them. I don't want it to be all 'me-me-me!' so I've brought in the views, opinions and experience of a wide range of people I've come into contact with since my diagnosis. They will add context to my story, as well as offering useful insights, thoughts, advice and information about the treatment – in all senses of the word – of people with life-changing or life-threatening conditions.

PART TWO

RIPPLES AND REFLECTIONS

In this section of the book I want to give context to my story in terms of the decade that has passed (at the time of writing) since my diagnosis, and what I have learned about myself and my condition since that day in September 2006. I also want to introduce the voices of others; friends, work colleagues and professionals who were there on my journey from diagnosis onwards and who can shed light not just on my experience, but theirs too. Few people experience a life-changing diagnosis wholly alone and those who are by their side, in whatever capacity, need to have a voice. This is important because it helps others understand what is involved when such a diagnosis is made, and how it creates the ripple effect which has so much bearing on what happens – or doesn't happen – next. If you're recently diagnosed with a life-changing condition and are wondering what to do, or you're close to someone who has, these pages are for you. Hopefully they will help you and those around you, in whatever capacity, to understand some of the feelings being experienced and what might be done to assist. I will address primarily the person who has been diagnosed, for no other reason than to not have to keep writing 'you/your partner/ friend/carer' all the time! Of course, everything that's said is useful for partner/friend/carer as well; if that's you, please keep reading and you your will glean plenty of practical advice and information.

So, the diagnosis has been given and as well as reeling from the shock, you're having to weigh up your future options. Suddenly, your life is limited – and not necessarily in the most obvious way. You may become less physically mobile or face potential issues in the workplace. You may not be able to participate fully in sport or other recreational activities. You may have difficulties getting life insurance or being able to drive. You may face significant side effects from the medication you've been prescribed or from other forms of treatment you're receiving. You might be tormented by mental ill health – most likely depression and/or anxiety – that have never previously troubled you. You might find that people you knew as friends or lovers suddenly become 'exes'. You might face stigmatisation, prejudice and scorn. Life-changing diagnoses aren't labelled as such for any reason.

BUT – where there is life, there is hope. And while you may be feeling that everything is stacked against you, the truth is that you – and you alone – have the power to change how you react to what has happened to you. In my experience of running groups for those newly diagnosed, people tend to fall into two camps: victims and survivors. And while you may feel that your life experiences and the way you process events leads you naturally down the dark path to depression and resignation, the truth is that you can choose whether you will be a victim or a survivor.

If you're the latter, you will have a better outlook on how to process your diagnosis and where to progress from this point. Maybe your first step was to pick up this book. If so, I can bet that it won't be the only thing you're reading; if you're a survivor you will be finding out as much as you can about your diagnosis and what it means for you. The survivor is the person who says, 'I'm going to deal with this. It won't dictate to me'. It involves a degree of fight; fighting against your condition, the system, your own body, what's in your head. It's a hard and all-consuming fight, but it's a fight worth having if you're on the survivors' side.

When I was first diagnosed I could have easily gone down the path of depression and despair. And I did. In truth, I was already on that path before the diagnosis of HIV. All the unexplained health problems I'd been having were really getting me down, plus the fact that I was approaching fifty and was beginning to have the usual, 'What is my life about?' thoughts. And yet, as I've described, when the diagnosis came I had a sense of relief, in that at least I knew there was something physically wrong with me and that I wasn't going mad. Still, there were plenty of times when I didn't feel like dragging my head from up off the pillow and facing a new day knowing what I knew about my health. I must thank Richard, my partner, and Dean Thomson, my community nurse, for not allowing this to happen.

RICHARD HOAD

For me, it was very important that Roland didn't become a victim. I said, "The one thing I can't cope with is that if you say, 'I can't work any more, I'm staying at home'." That would have broken our relationship. I'm not sure I could have had respect for somebody if they didn't at least try. And he kind of agreed with that. It was one of the important bits we needed to get done although it was hard for him to go back to work. I know some people who haven't worked since the day they were diagnosed, and I think it's a downward spiral. He's achieved a lot in the last ten years which he wouldn't have if he'd pulled the drawbridge up.

The role I took on was making sure he was cared for. I spoke to the doctors. I looked after his medication, his food, everything. He wasn't in a position to take it all in. When the consultant told me the diagnosis, I was shocked. I don't think

I thought about me, I just thought about him. Emotionally it was that weekend which was the worst for me, because I was unaware of what it all meant. The last person I knew that had died of AIDS was in '87 or '88, so I only had that as my single reference point. Then, there was no medication, nothing, so I was out of touch in terms of what could be done. I found that weekend difficult. Roland was sleeping most of the time, not able to get up or do anything. For me, the dishes needed washing as usual. It was probably my lowest point, not knowing what it all meant.

The biggest release for me was that first meeting with the consultant. She was a very nice lady and she said to us that with the advances in medication Roland would live a normal life like anybody else. And for me, having this reassurance was when and where the concern stopped. 'OK,' I thought, 'he might die a couple of years younger because of the medication or he might get run over by a bus, but there is no reduction in his life span from being HIV positive'. For me that was a great turning point. I'm an optimistic person anyway but up to that moment I was worried. Although it was rough for him with the various drugs he was taking, the side effects and things like shingles. That was a long period of hardship for him, and maybe a bit for me but only in terms of the effect it had on our relationship and what we could do. He'd often be ill and despite everything managed to get through work, but be out of it at weekends. So we didn't do much.

DEAN THOMSON

I was a community nurse in primary care when I met Roland. One of the clinics I was attached to was the one which Roland was referred from. He had received a positive diagnosis two weeks previously. He was concerned that he and his partner weren't managing well and adjusting to the diagnosis. Physically he was quite run down at the time. He had been suffering for ages with a variety of physical ailments. He attended with Richard and they both were still quite shell-shocked and getting used to the situation. In my time, in response to such diagnoses I've seen everything from furniture flying across rooms to people becoming withdrawn, potentially suicidal or just shutting down. At the time we called this stage 'pre-post-test counselling', which gauged how people responded to results.

After two weeks following diagnosis we'd normally be seeing some indications of an individual picking themselves up and taking steps forward about how they will manage with a positive result. Roland wasn't throwing chairs – we weren't at that stage – but if ten is throwing chairs and one is standing on a bridge we were looking about three or four in his case. He had grasped what he'd been told but wasn't addressing it emotionally, and physically he was still under par, so he was having to manage that as well. My best impression of Roland was that the shock had really knocked him off his feet. The one analogy I have used in my career is that when you get a diagnosis of HIV it is like being hit by a train. You fly through the air and hit the ground, and at some stage you have to get up. Roland had hit the ground but he wasn't able to get up. It's the same with any terminal diagnosis; it's a life-changing experience. And the double barrel was that it was also life changing for Richard and their relationship together. They had been making plans to marry at that point, then something came along which had a significant impact on relationships and families.

Dean is right. At first, the shock is enormous and all-encompassing. In my case, it was life-threatening, as people diagnosed late have a ten-fold increased risk of death within a year of HIV diagnosis compared to those diagnosed promptly ('Promotion for Sexual and Reproductive Health and HIV: Strategic Acton Plan for 2016-2019' Public Health England). That said, if and when you move out of the danger zone it's how you look at it in the aftermath that counts. I am grateful that Richard and Dean combined to bully me to not go down the victim route as I could have done quite easily. One of things Dean said to me early on was, "You're not recreating *Philadelphia*!" (1993 film starring Tom Hanks as a person dying from AIDS). Having people say those things is useful, they bring you up. That said, I think it's important there is an initial period of reflection and adjustment to the new circumstances.

RICHARD HOAD

At first we shut ourselves off from the world. We didn't tell anybody that we had not gone away on holiday. We told nobody about the HIV diagnosis. We told a few people about the encephalopathy – but that was only on a 'need to know' basis. We didn't go out at first, then we would start to make little day trips. For example, we'd drive to Windsor, sit in the car and read newspapers. Or we went to Poole Harbour. Once I'd managed to get him in the car he was OK. We did a couple of those trips where we drove somewhere, parked up and just ate our sandwiches, which got him out of the house. But that was it. Walking was too difficult.

For the first couple of months we just went down that path. It was just making sure he had everything he needed. We were at the hospital continuously for various things, including tests and check-ups, and it was about following whatever they said we needed to do. Everything was geared around that element, and it became our new normality.

In my case the impact was the severity of the condition and the fact that I'd had two weeks to live. Had I been diagnosed much earlier when I wasn't feeling unwell (or as unwell) then the impact might have been potentially less. In the UK, it is the case that 40% of diagnoses are defined as late, albeit that this has declined from 56% in 2005. ('HIV New Diagnoses, Treatment and Care in the UK 2015' Public Health England). When I deliver workshops for newly diagnosed people, I find they come for a whole range of reasons. Sometimes it's because they have been diagnosed for seven or eight years but haven't come to terms with it, particularly people who are isolated, have nobody with whom they can share this knowledge and are unable to process it. Obviously, the diagnosis has an impact on them, but they're not able to cope with that.

Had I been tested when I was feeling well, with no underlying problems, and the results had come back positive, I think my response would have been very different. Part of the way I reacted the way I did was because I was so unwell. My brain faculties were so screwed up that my overriding memory at the time is one of huge relief.

DEAN THOMSON

Even at that time there was still a lot of misinformation about HIV and AIDS and it was a case of trying to get the correct information into Roland's head, so he could ask questions in his own time, allowing him to open up to ask about what he could and couldn't do and what risks he was posing. We often don't look at and digest information unless it is relevant to us, and it is about accepting that relevance. Roland took his time taking ownership of the diagnosis. Once he did it was with a real degree of gusto and determination! He started running before he could walk. The point where he started engaging with the variety of support agencies and services was when I became concerned that he might be overdoing it. So my response was, "Slow down, and be comfortable with yourself before you influence or engage with other people who have their own take on what they are doing and which way they are going." He did things with gusto because I think he was overcompensating for that initial non-progression. That's slightly dangerous because if you haven't got a solid base of knowledge in your head or you're not quite comfortable with your diagnosis you can become heavily influenced by literature and groups out there.

RICHARD HOAD

In hindsight the diagnosis has given Roland something to hold on to because prior to being diagnosed it was a case of, 'I've reached fifty, what's the point of life, what's it all about?' Not in a suicidal way, but in a male menopausal way. And now he has a purpose. He's turned this into a positive thing. And when I think back to what it was in those first few days and weeks to where he is now, he deals with life as it is. I still remember having to rub the cream in for his shingles, rubbing his feet during the middle of the night to help ease the peripheral neuropathy, managing his showers and laundry to ensure that he didn't come into contact with soaps or washing powders that would further increase the irritation of his skin and so on. Those were tough times. Sure, he must still be careful if he gets a cold because he can go downhill quite quickly. Not to the point of death, obviously, but it takes longer for him to get back up. Other than those kind of issues, as he's got better and stronger, he's become more confident and taken over responsibility for his own treatment.

A life-changing diagnosis is the catalyst for very strong emotions. It also triggers the 'fight or flight' mechanism and after a few months I went into 'fight' mode. As Dean says, I really threw myself into doing something for others. Perhaps that was born of anger; anger at my various illnesses and the way they affected my life, and anger at my eventual diagnosis.

Overall, coming to terms with a life-changing diagnosis is about giving people back that belief in themselves. For me, it was finding the self-confidence to understand that while HIV is an important factor in my life and can't be ignored, it doesn't define me. I am not HIV. I am Roland. I happen to be living with HIV. It's very important to strike that balance. When you feel that loss of control, you feel disempowered and personal empowerment is vital.

Dr Alli Beardall was my consultant during that initial stage. Her perspective from a medical point of view is interesting, not least because patients rarely get to hear the personal views of those caring for them. Alli and I became friends and I hold her in high regard because of the empathetic way she listened and responded to my worries, fears and needs. I consider her a life-saver.

DR ALLI BEARDALL

To be fair, I don't remember every person I've treated but Roland is one and at that time, luckily, we had the triple antiretroviral (ARV) treatment and even though things were at the early-ish stage we could be an awful lot more positive than five years previously. But with Roland's particular condition there wasn't an awfully big body of evidence that the ARVs were going to wave a magic wand. Nowadays we know that putting people on ARV tends to resolve the problem and we can be more positive than we were before, but at that time encephalopathy was an AIDS-defining illness that shook people to the core and made them very worried about their life expectancy. Roland effectively had the AIDS diagnosis and having that was the thing people took the greatest time to adjust to because they'd seen friends die of AIDS. And yet, at the time Roland was diagnosed, we had a lifeline because of ARV.

Roland was an absolute champion and although he was shocked and horrified by the whole diagnosis he put his head down, worked at it and did everything he could possibly do to assist his recovery. It was a tough time and I think the hardest part was adjusting to the diagnosis. We are of a certain era and I think he found it hard to shake off the thought he had an AIDS-defining illness and how it equated with what he'd seen in other people. But he stuck to the tablet-taking regime, and back then the tablets weren't easy to take. The side effects were pretty horrendous. When Roland was diagnosed he had to take the meds at exactly the same time every day and because availability was so variable, there was no forgiveness in the regime.

As I mentioned, Alli was a wonderful listener and always gave me an hour per appointment so we could really go over the issues. I doubt that consultants have so much time now, but being able to dig in to what was bothering me, and how I might tackle it, was crucial.

At that time, it was part of clinical practice to spend a lot of time with our patients. As clinicians we were performing an all-round role, helping the patients come to terms with diagnosis. We fought to keep our lengthy appointment times with our patients and perhaps we shouldn't have done really, but HIV was a hugely devastating diagnosis – a real turning point. We fulfilled a number of roles; psychological, counselling, everything, and I feel very privileged to have gone through having an entirely in-patient based group of people to seeing this transform to out-patient based. To be a part of that was amazing. It was really our vocation. Way back when, we called it 'HIV counselling', now we call it 'HIV discussion' because ultimately if you were diagnosed then HIV had certain life expectancy, there were problems with insurance, workplace issues – all these things. Now, if you're diagnosed in good time you can have a normal life expectancy and consequently there is a huge drive to chase people who remain undiagnosed. The whole idea behind promoting HIV testing is no longer that it's a witch-hunt, it is totally treatable – so get tested.

I think the general thoughts or stigma or ideas around HIV have changed enormously. Going back, the whole 'hush hush, don't tell anyone, don't tell your GP' was so prevalent and now there is a big push towards GP communication and 90% of HIV patients are in GP correspondence. From the Black African point of view there are still huge stigmas because culturally people don't want to admit to being HIV, and every sub-Saharan country has different cultural issues. But even that situation has improved, though the sub-Saharan populations are still the hardest to deal with because of huge denial and an incredible suspicion of Western medicine. A lot still visit witch doctors and healers. They are probably now the biggest target group, because they are the group most undiagnosed. It used to be gay men, but their numbers have dropped recently and people are saying that's because of PrEP (Pre-Exposure Prophylaxis) but we will wait and see.

Slowly and surely, for all the at-risk groups things have improved enormously but there have been five or so years, particularly among the gay population, where an element of irresponsibility has crept in and is very evident. It is difficult to say that, with an overall drop in gay HIV diagnoses, but there has been an era of complacency which I think everyone has been aware of. For quite a while we've had Post Exposure Prophylactics (PEP) as well, giving four weeks of ARV therapy if you think you've been exposed. It is good to see the numbers dropping but I don't think it's anything to do with attitude.

Talking of which, I think people with a positive mental attitude like Roland have a greater chance of a better outcome living with HIV, as opposed to those who didn't run with it, and therefore didn't do so well. There are different psychologies and different hard wiring, of course, and there are people who genuinely cannot cope and never do. In that sense Roland has been an absolute champion; he is one of the most amazing people I've ever met.

DISCLOSURE - HOW, WHEN AND WHY

A big issue for me, and anyone else with HIV, is that of disclosure. And disclosure is such an ugly word, implying that there is always a big secret that has to be kept hidden. So let's use 'tell' instead. Whom do you tell, when do you tell and how do you do it so that its impact is minimised, both on you and the person whom you're telling? It's a thorny issue: some people never tell at all, except to those to whom they feel it is essential (medical people and the like) while others take to social media to declare their status to the world. Of course, there are positives and negatives in both approaches and as everyone is different there is no 'right' or 'wrong' way to approach it. Below are some thoughts on the subject…

DEAN THOMSON

One of the dangers of taking too much ownership of your status is the desire to tell as many people as possible about it. In the early 1990s, when I first started off in HIV care, we were constantly advised that the minute you tell someone you can't untell them and I always advocated caution and thought before disclosing a diagnosis to any party. I still remember one of the first guys with HIV I nursed at the London Hospital and his mum came from Ireland to visit. We'd prepared everything, and she'd flown in to visit this young lad in his early 20s. I brought her into the room where her son was hooked up to a machine and she didn't even take her coat off. She just stood at the end of the bed and said, "Never come home, never contact us." And then she walked off the ward. We had to pick up the pieces there, but it certainly wasn't an isolated case. I've had people being thrown out of rental accommodation for disclosing their status. They've been standing on the lawn with the landlord shouting at them. You may not encounter this much in London now, but in rural areas it can still be an issue. So I always advocate thinking seriously before you tell anyone. Of course, the situation for people diagnosed with HIV has changed; legislation is in place and we've seen attitudes towards HIV change in work and accommodation situations. You are more protected now, but in social situations we still see problems with families and relationships. It's the emotional link. People don't realise how much it can hurt being rejected.

I still remember a couple in their sixties, where one partner had kept his positive diagnosis from his mother, who was in her eighties. Yet she was picking up on the deterioration in her son's health and the couple actually celebrated when they received a HIV-related cancer diagnosis because now he was able to say to his mother, 'I have cancer'. And that was more acceptable for her to take on board. She had met the partner and had accepted there was a male friend, but it was never discussed that there was a relationship there. So these issues around disclosure do crop up.

Disclosure is all about the ripple effect. Once you drop a stone into the pond you can't manage what happens, and how far the ripples spread. You ask one person to keep it to themselves and inevitably it won't happen. That's just human nature, because people want to share it with someone. And sometimes the ripples are completely unexpected, and often they don't stop. The consequences of throwing that stone are different for everyone, and the action brings up issues for other people. However, you can't control that or take responsibility for them. For me, being open about my status is liberating and empowering, but it's also about recognising there are those ripple effects and being aware that you don't know how far the ripple will go. Personally, I'm now perfectly open about it. I write about it, I speak about it, I tell people. And for me it's that circular argument that there is still fear and mythology and stigma about HIV and AIDS because people who live with it don't talk about it. And when people don't talk about it the fear and sigma created by mythology and ignorance remain. So there is a cycle until we break it, and people can feel capable and able to say, "I'm living with it, so what? Apart from that I'm just like anyone else." But yes, you have to be discerning in some cases. In part, for me at least, some of this comes from my sexuality. For a long time I kept quiet about the fact that I was gay and very often it felt as though I was walking in shadows. I only came out at work when I joined the FCO and had to go through security procedures, so Richard had to be declared. And by then, I didn't see any reason why I shouldn't be open about it. But until 1990 the FCO wouldn't officially employ gay men. It did, of course, but they were red-tagged in secret files because they were deemed to be a security risk. When I was diagnosed, and I was able to deal with it, I decided that I'd walked in enough shadows and wouldn't walk in any more. I wasn't going to hide this.

However, telling is a hugely difficult, complicated area and is one of the big issues we spend a lot of time discussing in newly diagnosed groups. If you are already in a relationship with someone, straight or gay, and you are diagnosed, do you tell your partner and if so, how do you tell them? Inevitably, it's such a personal decision. The 2015 People Living with HIV Stigma survey identified that more than 15% of respondents had not told anybody about their HIV. Around three in five of the respondents felt well supported when sharing their status with family and friends but 12% of the participants had decided not to apply for, or turned down, employment or promotion due to their status.

I wouldn't want to say there is a right or wrong way of doing it and my situation was different to many other people's situations, in that it was my partner who told me about my diagnosis, not a medical professional.

Had it been the other way around, however, how would I have approached it? I would like to think that I would have done it as Richard did it, with love and care and concern, and support. But I think many other people wouldn't be so fortunate and I have worked with people whose relationships have broken down because of this. And in relationships where one person is diagnosed, their partner goes for the test and they are also diagnosed positive, the question arises of who gave it to whom, and in what circumstances? And does it matter?

RICHARD HOAD

I hadn't really thought I could be infected, to be honest. My concern was that because I knew I'd come into our relationship negative, if I had been infected how would that affect Roland's mental state? I was tested, it was negative and so we didn't have to go down that road.

I never really hit the blame button. My concern was, 'Is he going to survive?' I never once thought he was unfaithful, and maybe that comes from my sense that if he had been, I don't know if I'd have been that bothered. For me, there is a difference between love and sex. So if for whatever reason he had done something sexually I wouldn't have seen it as a betrayal of our relationship of the kind you might get with a straight male/female scenario.

I think I thought we were strong enough that if he had dabbled it wouldn't have affected the relationship. So that never even occurred to me. I didn't doubt our future was together. I remember him saying to me, "Please don't throw me out." And I said, "Why would I do that? There is no need for that at all." I think he thought I was going to be more upset than I was. This was our home, it never occurred to me, but he did pick up on it and said it often for the first few months.

Richard and I are in a monogamous relationship and the medical professionals were able to identify that I had been infected before I even met Richard. But there is that thing around, 'If you're positive and I'm negative you must have caught it from risky behaviour with someone else'. So there is potential for an enormous amount of stress around this issue, both within established relationships and new ones too. If the HIV positive person is single and is looking for a relationship, the question that crops up time and again is, 'I've met someone I quite like, when should I tell them?' And very often we hear that the HIV positive person has been honest and told – and that's been the end of the relationship before it's barely begun. Those of us who are HIV positive are often asked, 'Are you clean?' The implication being, of course, that if you're 'not clean', i.e. you are HIV positive, then you must be 'dirty'. Those who are affected by cancer, of whatever type, are never asked if they are 'clean'. Today, many people experience cancer, either as a patient or as a relative or friend of someone with cancer, and many people survive it, so we are more open about it. Yet, a 2017 University of Bristol (School of

Social and Community Medicine) study found that the expected age at death of a twenty-year-old HIV patient starting antiretroviral therapy (ART) after 2008, with a low 'viral load' (the term used to describe the amount of HIV in your blood; i.e. the higher viral load the more chance you have of becoming ill because of HIV, and the lower the viral low the higher the chance you have of becoming 'undetectable') and after the first year of treatment, was seventy-eight years – similar to the general population. So why should such a person be 'clean' or 'dirty'? Part of the reason, I think, goes back to a Victorian state of mind around three big taboos: sex, homosexuality, death. And HIV touches all three.

I remember how cancer awareness days were always big news at the Foreign Office. There would be a bake sale, or a ribbon sale or a sponsored something or other. All great, and all raising money for excellent causes. Yet when I went around with a collecting tin on World AIDS Day I came away with £12 and a button. It's not surprising – HIV and AIDS affect a very small population in the UK compared to cancer – but it is disappointing. This despite statistics that reveal that the overwhelming majority of people in the UK (79%) agree that people with HIV deserve the same level of support and respect as people with cancer ('HIV – Public Knowledge and Attitudes, 2014: A study for the National AIDS Trust' by Ipsos MORI). Perhaps private feelings don't always translate into public support.

So yes, telling people you have HIV can be complex indeed. Much depends on the relationship you have with the person you're potentially disclosing to. The issue arises quite often with telling parents. Personally, I made the decision not to tell my mother as I did not want to add to the burdens of her old age. But I did tell my brother and the reaction was negative in the extreme, at least at first. I can think of specific examples of people on newly diagnosed courses who've had very a close relationship with parents and actually want their support, but are concerned about how their parent(s) might react, from the one who gets very angry ('How could you be so stupid?', 'What were you up to?!') to those who become overly anxious and concerned that you will die before them. But again, I don't think it would be appropriate to generalise, as everyone's circumstances are unique.

My personal philosophy is that it's always best to be open and honest. If you want to tell someone, perhaps one of the best and easiest ways is to raise the subject of HIV and see how that person responds to it. Once you've gauged their reaction to the topic in general you can then judge how safe it feels to tell them about yourself. I find that when I have declared my status to someone and they haven't been in possession of the full facts I take that opportunity to educate and inform, not lecture. 'This is what is happening'; 'This is the current state of affairs' or 'You might find it useful to know this.'

Maddy Coulson and Suzanne Nicolson have been friends of mine and Richard's for a long time. They were the first friends I told my status to.

MADDY COULSON

Suzanne and I were planning our civil partnership and Roland was helping me to prepare all the flowers, so we were in their lounge doing this. We were a week away from the date, and I wanted him to read a poem at the ceremony. There was obviously something bothering him and then he sat back and said, "I have something to tell you." He looked so serious; my heart was in my mouth and he just came out with it. He hadn't been well for some time, no one knew what it was, and it had gone on and on and we were all very worried about him. So he came straight out with it.

My first reaction was shock because it wasn't something on my radar. We'd thought of all kind of conditions and I don't know why I hadn't thought of HIV, but I just hadn't. It never crossed our minds. I was just so shocked, and I said, "I didn't expect that. We need a hug here." So we hugged and cried, as you would, and then he said, "How do you feel about it? Is it a worry for you?" Well of course it wasn't, not at all. From my point of view, I had no personal fears of HIV. Back in the early 80s one of my closest friends worked on the AIDS research team at the Royal Free Hospital in London and I learned more about AIDS and HIV than most people would. Even so, I was shocked because it hadn't crossed my mind. We just talked about it and Roland said he hadn't told anyone else other than Richard, and Richard was very concerned about anyone knowing because it's something you have to be ready for, and he was worried Roland wasn't ready for it. I then told Susie when she came to pick me up.

SUZANNE NICOLSON

I was out working and when I arrived to pick Maddy up both she and Roland were crying. So I realised something was quite serious and once we were in the car Maddy told me Roland was unwell. I thought it was cancer at first until she told me it was HIV. At first I was shocked because I thought, 'Roland is not that type'. My immediate thought was that HIV usually affected promiscuous people and in the context of Roland this didn't make sense. After the initial shock I realised that HIV can affect anyone of course, and I became extremely protective of Roland. He read a poem at our civil partnership and halfway through he burst into tears. We stood beside him and held his hand,

and it was a case of, 'We're there for you, mate, no matter what'.

I am naturally a protective person, and even though I know Richard is looking after Roland I still keep an eye on him. Many people have this condition, but I do feel people are still frightened of it. I used to work in the care industry doing assessments for people who needed stairlifts and I came across a few people with HIV/AIDS. My own team of guys were often scared to go into houses because of AIDS, and would be shocked if I stopped for a cup of coffee with the infected person.

I think that even now, anyone with HIV still has to be cautious about who they tell. The world still isn't quite ready for gay people, there is still a stigma around being gay in some areas and I would say, 'To begin with, heed on the side of caution'. When I was working I was nervous of telling my new boss I was in a gay relationship, and Maddy was actually forced out of a job because she was gay and that was in the late 90s. There are still things that people are very uncomfortable about, and plenty of narrow minds out there. Education is what is needed, particularly around families because families really can make or break a situation.

MADDY COULSON

Following Roland's diagnosis, the only thing I wanted do was to wrap him up in cotton wool and tell him it would be alright. Being HIV positive is NOT a death sentence. I knew enough about it to know that. But I did know that he would have to be placed on very stringent medication and monitored but I had absolutely no idea to what extent and how it might work. The situation as regards medication is changing all the time anyway, and this area has vastly improved even from when Roland was diagnosed.

That said, I didn't honestly feel a great deal of relief knowing he was HIV positive because I knew enough that he would have a huge uphill struggle and the illness itself is still undefined, among the general public at least. If you're diagnosed with cancer everyone knows what cancer is, and about its different types. HIV is still so under-publicised in terms of what people go through and I did wonder whether for Roland, it would open up a can of worms. He and Richard have great friends who would be able to handle that type of news, but I felt family wouldn't be told. I worried for him about telling people.

Support-wise, initially we asked Roland what he would have to do and what medication he was on. He explained that he'd have to take it at so many hourly intervals and when we went on holiday with Roland and Richard after our civil partnership, every time his watch alarm went off we all said simultaneously, "Roland, your medication!" So there were the three of us, in our cack-handed way, trying to make sure he never forgot his medication. We tried to normalise it in some ways and thereafter, when Roland had a bad turn (which he frequently did in the early years) we understood why and that meant he didn't have to go into any great explanation. We knew the background and they knew they could turn to us.

For anyone else in the position of being friends or relatives of someone with HIV I would say that it's important to show solidarity, to not shy away and to ask questions. A lot of people won't know much about the condition; they'll have heard about it but it's likely they're not up-to-date with developments. Rather than think, 'Oh God I can't talk about this' and cross the road, it's far better to be open and positive and not to be afraid to ask questions because a person who has this diagnosis probably needs to talk.

SUZANNE NICOLSON

It's made me very close to Roland because I feel honoured he chose to tell us so early and because I feel we learned so much from this. It's not just about HIV or AIDS; there are other life-changing diseases people have, and now we don't judge them in quite the same way because you know someone who has or had it. Maddy's dad passed away with vascular dementia, and we had hard times but learned a lot from that. Roland's condition is hidden to a large extent. A lot of our friends still don't know. We've told some people with his permission but with the rest we just don't talk about it. As human beings, do we tell everyone about every condition we have? No, of course not, so why make a big deal about this one? Some people might need to know, but otherwise...?

Having told Maddy and Suzanne so that, should anything happen to me, Richard would have people 'in the know' that he could turn to, Richard also wanted me to have that same safety net. So I also told old friends Pip and David Ashton. I am godparent to their three children (despite being an atheist!) and I knew once I told them that Pip and David would understand what was happening and be supportive. Additionally, Pip is an intensive care nurse.

DAVID ASHTON

We'd been concerned for a while because Roland kept being unwell and obviously we were very upset when we heard he had the condition, but he'd had time to rationalise it and could tell us matter-of-factly. It was still a shock, though, because he had been in a relationship a long time and so we didn't expect that to be the reason for his constant illnesses.

PIP ASHTON

I believe we probably were one of the first people Roland told. I remember he invited us to dinner, which wasn't unusual at all. He sort of sat us down after dinner and said that he had something he needed to tell us. I just remember being quite shocked and worried for him, I suppose. My concern was more about him than anything else.

One of the things that I felt was a bit stupid for not having picked up on it before. Partly because he had been unwell and he had encephalopathy, which is actually an AIDS-defining disease; if somebody comes in with that, then you would automatically test for HIV/AIDS. I felt stupid that I had missed it. I felt I should have picked it up. I also felt – and Roland has since said that it wasn't the case – that perhaps he had told me what was wrong with him expecting at that point I would pick up on what that meant before he needed to come out and say it bluntly, before he actually put it into words. As a nurse I should have picked up what it meant.

We were completely shocked, but other than that I really don't think it's made that much difference to the way we view him. It certainly hasn't made any difference to the way we've had contact with him. I suppose the only thing that I'm a little warier of is if we've got stinking colds or are really unwell ourselves. Then I would tend to avoid coming into contact with Roland, especially if he's under the weather himself at the time. So if we were due to meet up and I was not on top form, then

I would contact him and say that we're not well and 'Would it be better if we avoid you?' Whereas with anyone else I probably wouldn't do that; if I was feeling under the weather but not unwell enough that I could still go out, I would still go. But with him I tend to think 'Hang on a moment, is this the best thing?'

As a friend, is there a right and a wrong way to take news like this? I'm not sure there is, because everyone is different, and everybody's reaction is going to be very different. I think it's important to understand and empathise with the way this might affect you; that it makes very little difference, and it's not going to change anything as it stands. Obviously if the disease progresses then we're looking at a different story.

I think for somebody who's going to be telling somebody else, it's about being able to give the information that's needed. When giving any bad news, people will only hear what they're ready to hear. Almost whatever you're going to say, if they're not ready to hear it, they won't hear it. The other thing is to be prepared to take questions. That was one of the things with Roland that we talked about with the children; he wanted to answer any of the questions they might have and to give as honest an answer as he could.

Also, I think you have to frame the disclosure to the person you're telling it to, and at their level. Then as you can gather the way they are understanding, you can increase or decrease the amount of information you give. Sometimes you start almost gently; you introduce the idea and people will either pick up on it or they won't. If you realise they're not picking up on it, gradually you have to become blunter. Start with general hinting at what you're trying to say, and hope that they ask the questions, and then become more candid.

DAVID ASHTON

If you're given a diagnosis like this from a person you're close to, I think it's very important to remember the person you knew from before they were ill. You liked that person before and you'll continue to like them now. Nothing has changed personality-wise, so don't treat them any differently. I also think it's important to do your research. Find out about your friend's condition, discover what it means for them and understand the effects of the medication they'll be on. The more you understand, the better you will understand what that person is going through. And if there is a partner involved, be there for them too. We're as close to Richard as we are to Roland and we were equally supportive of him as they went through this.

I also told early on my friend Joyce Franks, whom I've known for more than thirty years. For me, telling people I had HIV was like coming out as gay all over again. Joyce picks up on this:

JOYCE FRANKS

I can remember when he told me he was gay. He'd come over for supper at my house and he just said, "I want to tell you something – I'm gay." And I said, "Yes, I thought possibly you were." That was it. It didn't bother me one way or the other, and I knew when he felt that he could trust me enough to tell me, he'd tell me. I thought it was incredibly brave of him. Especially at that time, because of what was going on in the 80s.

I think it was over dinner again that he told me he had HIV. I knew that he had been incredibly ill, I mean really quite seriously ill. It was about that time that he told me and in all honesty, I was more concerned about the encephalopathy than I was about the HIV. With a nursing background I knew how serious encephalopathy could be. I was scared for him more with regard to the encephalopathy than the HIV at that particular time, although I knew HIV was very serious.

And yet, he was always ambitious in a very positive way, he always wanted to make the best of what he had and to improve and to get promoted into a different area. But his drive is much stronger now I think. He is much more confident in himself. I think he knows himself now and if you don't like him then that's your problem not his. He says what he wants to do, and he goes out and does it. I think that is probably because of having HIV and seeing from the inside what needs to be done rather than the outside. He will do what he says he's going to do, or he'll have a jolly good try and if he doesn't succeed then OK, but he tried.

Maddy Coulson's comment about people crossing the street is spot-on. It's usually a metaphor, of course, for a conversation other people would not rather have with you (though no doubt some people do actually cross the street to avoid someone they know with a rather awkward illness!) And if there is a conversation, it's quite often on the lines of, "Oh, but you look so well!" or "You'd never guess there's anything wrong with you!" or "Oh dear, I'm so sorry…" I try to take such comments with the misplaced sympathy with which they're delivered but for me, the best response to a disclosure is, "I'm sorry to hear that. How are you?" It's a simple as that, and it gives the person living with the condition a chance to talk about the diagnosis – or not, as the case may be. People who've heard someone is HIV positive or has cancer very often agonise over their response, and inevitably over-complicate it. But it needn't be complicated. These things can happen to anyone. Even you!

LOOKING FOR SUPPORT

Soon after diagnosis I reached out to find the kind of support I thought I'd need among people who genuinely understood what I was going through, i.e. people in the same situation as me. In short, what we might term the 'HIV community'.

But what is the 'HIV community'? Well, it certainly isn't one amorphous thing. There are those people who have been recently diagnosed, and understand that while they will have to take medication every day (and keep an eye on their health a little more closely than others might need to) their life expectancy is near-normal. There are also those who have lived with HIV for many years and have the battle scars of ill health, unemployment, relationship breakdowns and on-going stigma to prove it. And in many ways, never the twain shall meet. The younger, newly diagnosed group are often seen as not giving enough respect to the generation from the 1980s who've had it tough, while the veterans see the 'one pill a day' group as irresponsible at best, reckless at worst. Certainly, there are issues around rising levels of HIV infection among younger men who engage in 'chemsex' (and men already diagnosed who are into chemsex). Wikipedia defines chemsex as the consumption of drugs to facilitate sexual activity and refers to a subculture of recreational drug users who engage in high-risk sexual activities under the influence of drugs within groups. In 2014 a Positive Voices survey of HIV-positive patients attending thirty HIV clinics in England and Wales, presented at the Conference on Retroviruses and Opportunistic Infections (CROI 2016), has found that nearly a third (29%) of gay male patients reported engaging in 'chemsex'.

Like everything, there are generalisations and the battle lines are nowhere nearly so defined in many cases. But it is true that the 'HIV community' or even the 'gay community' are lumped together, whereas any community has sub-groups, diverse needs, conflicting interests, etc. etc. Surprisingly, I have found some prejudice against the gay HIV community from the gay non-HIV community on the basis that being HIV is somehow connected with drug-taking or promiscuity. I hope that the HIV community, such as it exists, holds no prejudices against anyone with HIV; straight, gay, black or white. Again, one cannot generalise.

Esther, a friend of mine, is a straight black woman living with HIV in London. I met her in 2014 on a course I was running.

ESTHER WILLIAMS

I'd been to various meetings and become really interested in the issues around HIV. I became involved with UK-CAB in September 2014 and then in November I met Roland. He was just really sweet, a really nice guy. He came across as very competent, just someone who had their stuff together. I warmed to him immediately. There were a few 'chaotic' people there during that weekend – at the time I was thinking, 'I don't want to be put in the same group as IV drug users or sex workers'. So there was this whole blame thing going on from my part. At the time, I didn't understand the human rights aspect of things. So, I was just like 'I don't want to be put into this group'. Even though, the truth of it is it doesn't actually matter. I discovered that fairly early on about this, talking to Roland. He said, "The fact is that you've got it and that's where we go from there. It doesn't really matter how it happened, it's just that it's happened, so deal with it." It took me a while to get over this, and understand it. I had to adjust my mindset, because I realised that was internalised stigma and I couldn't buy into that. That was just as dangerous. Though I guess I was meeting people I wouldn't naturally get on well with and I didn't want to be around such people if our only link was that. The last thing you want is to be defined by an illness which is manageable.

TELLING IN THE WORKPLACE

This is a fiendishly tricky area for anyone with HIV, particularly those in otherwise excellent health. Should you tell your boss or your work colleagues? Do you really need to tell them? And if you decide to tell, what might be the likely effects of that disclosure? The first thing to remember (as I've said before) is that HIV does not define you. You are you – you are not HIV. You just happen to be living with it. If you don't think it's anyone else's business, and it's not going to interfere with your work, you aren't obliged tell your workplace. Remember that from the day you're diagnosed you're covered by the 2010 Equality Act, which makes it unlawful to discriminate against anyone with HIV. This applies to workplaces, as well as education and customer services, which means that if you do share your status and you suffer discrimination as a result, you can take action in the civil courts.

There are, however, certain advantages in disclosing your status at work. Under the 2010 Act, one of the main areas concerning anyone with HIV (and, in fact, anyone with a disability which is what HIV is considered to be) is that you can request 'reasonable adjustments' – ways in which disadvantages can be removed so that you can work effectively. My own reasonable adjustments included, among other things, travelling to work outside the rush hour being offered a lower grade job whilst still being paid the higher grade salary and using audio voice recognition software. However, as I've detailed in my story there were issues and challenges in my place of work around my health which meant having fights of varying degrees of severity during periods when I felt least like fighting anything or anyone. Yet making the decision to tell my work colleagues was the best thing I did. When you have something like HIV the feeling of disempowerment, particularly at work when you're surrounded by 'healthy' colleagues (who might not be as healthy as they look, but even so!) can be overwhelming. I felt exactly this as I went through my various trials and tribulations. Attempting to restore that balance of power is important for the person living with HIV and when I did share at that lunchtime briefing, and got the reaction I got, I realised I had a voice that people were – and are – willing to listen to. That voice gives me the sense of empowerment I needed to move forward both professionally and personally. Having the rug pulled from under your feet is difficult. Suddenly your future has changed because your perspective of what your future may be has changed. You aren't the person you were, and that's difficult. Taking control of that situation can mean many things, and although there were blips I never regretted sharing my status with anyone at work. And statistics show that 67% of the public agree they would be comfortable working with someone living with HIV ('HIV – Public Knowledge and Attitudes, 2014: A study for the National AIDS Trust' by Ipsos MORI). But again, much depends on you and your situation. The same set of statistics also show that 37% agree with the statement 'My employer should tell me if one of my work colleagues is HIV positive'…

Having shared, and metaphorically plastered my name across the HIV banner in the FCO, I did have two colleagues who came to me who had been diagnosed and hadn't told anyone. They'd been diagnosed early on and weren't unwell. I also had a lovely woman who came to find me because her daughter had been diagnosed and was very ill in hospital. She wanted comfort and reassurance. And a colleague sought me out because he'd worked in a Far Eastern country and had had a local girlfriend. They were no longer together but she had contacted him because her brother was very ill with AIDS and, because homosexuality is illegal in that country, no treatment is available for people with HIV and AIDS. She was desperate to get medication. So this other chap and I, through embassy contacts, got some medication to her. They were drops in an ocean, but at least some good was coming from my disclosure.

That said, no one was ever openly hostile to me. And when I'm working with people who have experienced open hostility it makes me feel unworthy because I haven't had that experience. And I do wonder why I never had it. I wonder if it's because I have found this voice, this courage, this confidence to say, 'if you don't like it it's your problem, not mine'? I have no reason to need to hide it, whereas for other people who aren't so lucky, there may be a reason they need to hide it. If you are in the position where you feel you are forced to tell then it comes out in a different way, and possibly one in which you feel you have little control.

At the time of my diagnosis and subsequent disclosure Marta Nunez was my line manager. She is now a good friend. She has an interesting perspective of HIV in the workplace from a manager's point of view.

MARTA NUNEZ

When Roland joined, and I started to get to know him, I found him to be a great professional with a fantastic sense of humour. We got on very well. Sometimes we had different points of view, but he was always amicable. I knew how ill he was, and that he had had many tests which finally came the result that was HIV positive. I don't know how soon he told me after having received the result, but I think it was quite soon. Personally, I was devastated. Now of course I didn't show that: I said the usual things you say – "There are so many ways now that you can live with it." But personally, people I knew that had AIDS were now dead. I knew three people that had died. This was probably during the earlier days of the AIDS epidemic, and while I knew treatment had progressed since, I was still terribly sad and shocked about Roland.

In the context of work, managing the knowledge of his status was difficult because on the one hand I fully understood what he was going through, and on the other hand we as a department were going through a difficult time. That meant I had to play political games to save my team, but it put pressure on all of us. At that time Roland did whatever he was capable of doing but he was very ill. Sometimes it was either the medication he was taking, or that he seemed to have constant 'flu and respiratory problems. He looked ill and sometimes he couldn't make it to work.

I had to make sure that we were performing well. These were hard times for everybody. There were people having nervous breakdowns, going through depression, it was really sad. It was very sad for me as well at that time. I remember after a while of being there I had to start having counselling; the pressure was immense.

We tried to reschedule some of Roland's management tasks, but rumours were going around about him. My boss said that it was not the right moment to inform people, but I remember being in a situation where a colleague said to me, "Well look, this doesn't sound right, what does he really have?" Of course I couldn't say, but she was very suspicious. She was saying that whatever he has, it has to be communicated, because we were sharing PCs and general office space. It was very uncomfortable, this opinion, and Roland didn't know about this, so I said, "HR has been informed, Occupational Health knows about it. So if they haven't made any recommendations it's because it's not contagious. You have to be assured that the Foreign Office is not going to put anybody at risk." Without her saying, I knew what she was thinking, and she knew what I was implying without mentioning it.

On the one hand what we really needed was more input from Roland, because the team was already under a lot of pressure. However, I knew that what he could do was limited because his illness had affected some cognitive aspects of his brain. I was aware that there was a discussion going on about early retirement on health grounds and I was saying, "There is nothing much we can do at the moment. He probably will improve, and can I have more resources?" So in order to have those resources, I was told the only way that I could get some extra help was by writing that Roland could not deliver at this moment. I was made to write really awful letters. I had to say, "He's not delivering", "His health is impinging upon his productivity" and "There is an issue of how many times he has to go to the doctor or to look after himself when he doesn't feel well."

I understand the pressure Marta was under. When you're a manager in a situation like this you're often faced with such dilemmas and it's hard to know where your loyalties lie. Is it to the individual, to your team or to what your superiors are telling you to do? Workplace legislation around disability now goes some way to improving this situation for employees and managers alike, but as usual there is always room for improvement. We still haven't reached the stage where disclosure of HIV at work is regarded in the same way as a disclosure of cancer, or some other life-changing condition. It's interesting to read how Marta felt when I finally decided to 'come out', as it were, to my colleagues.

MARTA NUNEZ

At some moment we decided that it was the right time and so we gathered the team. This day was awful for me. I remember that I was late because I had a panic attack before arriving. I must have been like five or ten minutes late, which was very embarrassing. I thought maybe I would start to cry but I had to really compose myself and get there. I'd had no training in this and now I feel like I'd have benefited from some beforehand. I was very concerned about Roland; it was a difficult message to give to everybody. HR sent someone, but she was only an admin person, not someone trained in this kind of thing. She did what she could to facilitate it, but I would have much preferred to have a specialist there who could probably have facilitated it more effectively.

The reaction he got was very positive. People were incredibly moved, and they were really nice to him. We hugged him, the team reacted really well. It shows that they were all nice people. Some of them were very young, so maybe they were much more informed. I said to the woman who'd been asking about Roland's health, "Look, now you know, and this is in the hands of Occupational Health so stop it." Also, I said, "If you read the recent information you know how it can be caught, the illness, so come on."

Roland was brave; very, very brave. And if I had to go

through a similar thing again, I definitely would have demanded to have someone in that meeting who was a specialist on the topic. And I would have demanded to have counselling from them, and not end up me having to discuss things with my private counsellor. On a personal level, I've learnt a lot from Roland's experience. I've learnt about how difficult it is to deal with such conditions as a manager. I feel very guilty about writing those letters for instance, because I was exaggerating so we could receive more help. I was doing it for the right reason, and I was doing it because they were telling me it was the only way, otherwise they would not take it into consideration. All I wanted is for them to understand that extra help was needed and to keep Roland, to allow him to recover.

The following observations are from Anne Sylvester, whom I met a few years into my time at the Foreign Office. Anne was working as the Diversity Manager in Foreign Office Services and we worked on a few projects together. She was always a lively, bouncy person with a lovely informal way about her – she breathed life into what at times could be a stuffy organisation.

ANNE SYLVESTER

When I first met him, Roland was the chair of the Disability Action group, which was kind of struggling, from what I can remember. I knew he had a disability; I reckoned that he wouldn't have been the chair of DA if he hadn't! I could see from his spectacles that he was quite badly short sighted, but other than that I had no idea whatsoever. So we got to know each other, and I think there was a sort of professional respect between the two of us. The job for FCO diversity services adviser came up and Roland said, "What do you think?

Should I apply for it?" and I said, "I think you'd be absolutely perfect" and from then we got to work together far more, and we got to know each other a lot better. I realised that we came at things from a pretty similar angle because I had years of experience and he obviously had life experience. We would have a cup of coffee together and occasionally we'd go out and have a bite to eat and generally speaking, tear our hair out about how difficult it was to get anything done. We worked together on one or two projects, and eventually Roland decided to share his story with me. And I was just absolutely bowled over, (a) to be privileged to be told, and (b) to hear the story and how it had happened.

I wasn't shocked. I was surprised maybe, because I hadn't thought of it being anything as enormous as that. And having already worked with him, I was amazed how he managed to get himself on to the train and to work every day. It had obviously had a profound effect on the way he wanted to live his life. Roland and I have worked together on various presentations and we found that we work together very well. He's a consummate professional and he's a brilliant presenter. I think he realised that he had a safe ear in me, he's met my husband and the four of us have all socialised together, so there's a sort of trust and confidence about it, and between partners as well.

Anne knew that I was having some difficulties at work with one particular manager...the one who criticised my writing, not Marta.

I know there wasn't much empathy or sympathy towards his plight, it was just sort of 'get on with it' and 'stiff upper lip' as far as I can gather. I think he voluntarily took a down-grade in seniority. So, that had all kind of happened when

I knew him, and I think he was in a slightly better place, but probably still smarting about it. Then it happened again. He was labelled with all sorts of problems that he didn't have. A female manager used to talk about the fact that his writing skills weren't very good, and if you've ever seen the stuff that Roland can put down on paper then that really isn't the case. It might not have been in Foreign Office 'speak' but he wasn't a diplomat with a capital 'D'. He was failed really badly. Because of Roland's interest in the role, it should've been the time in his career that he really enjoyed, but was overshadowed by all of this going on in the background.

When he used to tell me about it I'd make sure to say that if he wanted to go through the grievance procedure that I would support him, but I really don't think he had the strength at the time to do it. He just sort of went ahead with all of the improvements suggested; go on a course, learn about this and that, have a mentor, but then of course again, with the Foreign Office rulings about career posts, the two years came and went. So again, I said "Well, look, I think you could use this to stay in the same post, and ask for it as a reasonable adjustment for your disability." But again, I think it was just too big a mountain.

So then Roland moved out and found a more supportive manager and had a better time. But at the bottom of it all there was a lot of unhappiness and when he got the chance to go, he took it.

I asked Anne what she considered is a good approach to managing anyone with a condition like HIV:

Well, the first rule of managing is to know what needs to be done. My opinion is that unless it's a newly diagnosed condition, most people are their own experts in their disability. My way to deal with it was to go and talk to the person and say, "How can we help you, what can we do, which is the best way to look at this?" Simple questions, not rocket science. And to try to gain their confidence, that actually I want to do the best for them so that they can achieve their full potential and we get the best out of them. At the end of the day, this means your business is doing better. If you engage properly with a person with a disability and you encourage them to fulfil their potential, they are more loyal, they stay longer and they are more productive.

If we're talking about disclosure and managing it so that it is easy and comfortable for everybody involved, again the first rule of a being a manager is that you should make it plain that this is what has happened, this is how we're going to deal with it and this is how we're going to behave. Most big organisations will have someone to deal with diversity, who should be the expert and be there on hand. That said, there has been a number of times I've had to get involved and stand between the person with the disability and the stroppy manager who either can't be bothered or hasn't got time or whatever, and say, "Well actually, you're going to listen to me, and you're going to do this", and explain why. And pointing out that there is legislation here that the manager could be falling foul of.

And I will say to people that in any form of diversity, complaints and wrong treatment nearly always come in from left of field – never from where you expect them. Often it's a curveball, and I always used to say, "Whatever it is, we can deal with it." If it's a quick fix, don't let it escalate because these things will go from nought to 50,000ft in three seconds.

On my own watch I had a particular manager of a department constantly trying to alter one woman's working patterns. Now these were the particular working patterns, including home-working and remote work that she'd been doing for a number of years. She'd never had any criticism on her annual report, and she produced the goods. The reason for her working pattern was that she had a severely disabled adult child. This manager tried to alter her working patterns, and I said, "Be very careful." She said, "What are you saying?" and I replied, "I am only advising you, that you are wide open to challenge and you can't alter someone's working conditions without a good reason." This woman said, 'She hasn't got a disability and said it was just about raising children." I said, "No it isn't, this is a lifetime responsibility for this woman." So, I told her all about a similar case and I said "Look, this woman will put in a grievance." This kind of attitude is harmful to everyone, it makes the air toxic, and nobody ever really wins at the end of the day.

Sure enough, the woman went off sick and put in a grievance. I had several meetings with this manager, with HR present. They consulted a solicitor and he quoted exactly the same legislation that I had quoted. Then our business partner, whom I knew quite well, said to this woman manager, "Well, Anne did point this out," and she said, "Anne's just a manager." The business partner said, "She might be 'just a manager', but she's managed a lot of disabled people, she's our diversity manager, she knows a lot about equality." Unfortunately, people don't always listen if it's not what they want to hear.

I first met Mary Brunton, an HR specialist and trainer with her own company, when we were working at the Foreign Office. She was my coach at the FCO during some of the difficult times there. Mary left to set up her own business, which includes delivering coaching and training to the FCO. I now work with her to do exactly the same thing. Mary has some interesting insights into what it takes to be open and honest about an HIV diagnosis in the workplace (and, for that matter, any other hidden disability).

MARY BRUNTON

Like anyone in a minority group who is willing to talk about what being in that minority group is like for them, what Roland brought specifically was visibility. He was willing to talk about it, willing to stand up and be counted, willing to say what is has been like for him. Roland has the ability to engage and be honest and for him to say, "This is the truth." It gives people an opportunity to be curious and brave, and to engage with these things. He does this through a combination of openness and visibility.

How do we encourage others to come forward and be visible? In my experience, there is a tendency for people who are in the roles such as Roland was – in Diversity, HR, that kind of thing – to be naturally more open and honest about their backgrounds. The trick is to find people in other areas of the business – so, for example, if we're talking about the Foreign Office we're perhaps looking for people in counter-terrorism or working out in some difficult location – doing jobs which co-exist with who they are. Their disability status isn't defining them, it's just part of who they are. These are the people we need to come forward and say, 'This is me, and it's fine'. Other people will get used to that, and eventually won't even think about it.

It is very difficult because disability status is the business of that person alone, and yet it's important to encourage other people to realise that the status of their colleague is just one thing about them. The aim is to get others to the point where disability status isn't the first thing they think when they think about their colleague.

So it's about asking people to be brave, to stand up and be counted. For example, I know someone who has mental health challenges and during Mental Health Awareness Week they organised a talk with all their colleagues about what it was like for them. They talked about what they did and what they needed from other people. They were brave, and the following day they felt completely different about their job and their colleagues. People came up to them and were understanding. So you encourage people by providing role models who are everyday people, just like the rest of us. And also, people who are in positions of authority or respected people. There are nowhere near enough of those standing up for disability awareness in public life.

Kate Nash is the Chief Executive of Purple Space, a unique networking and professional development hub for Chairs of disabled employee networks. I've known her since my time as Chair of the Disabled Employees Network at the Foreign Office and she has a lot of useful things to say about disability in the workplace, and why work is a vital way to regain confidence and self-esteem:

KATE NASH

I would say that the value of work to disabled people is critical. Life experiences such as disability or other health-related issues can leave you more isolated than other people. Life has thrown you a curveball and as you're navigating that stuff it is helpful to be engaged with others. Essentially, it's about staying in the game of life. Work drives everyone round the twist now and then, you have good times and bad times but mostly it keeps us in that game of existence. For people with disabilities there are barriers, including persuading employers to do things differently and introduce better working practices, and these external barriers are real. Also, there are internal barriers to face and a lot of these are about inner confidence. Issues such as eroded self-esteem and inner confidence can become neglected, as can navigating pity, which is a real issue for disabled employees. Disability and ill health is an experience that other people can't help but feel a degree of sadness, disappointment and pity towards. Pity is right at the edge of that range of emotions; it is corrosive and quite hard to navigate. It's difficult to hold your own at work and feel confident and sassy if all you're feeling is others' pity.

For disabled employees it's about noticing the hotspots – the times you feel a lack of confidence and identifying what you need to do to strengthen that. For example, Roland's ability to encourage individuals with HIV to notice how their confidence has been eroded is really essential and critical.

Disabled employees need to be able to bring their authentic selves to work, so they are who they are in the context of their job. They need to be able to share their truth as a human being, and to ask for workplace adjustments with ease and without too many questions. For their part, employers need to notice that there is a lot of human difference out there – that one size doesn't fit all – and be open to this with flexible working practices, adjustments needs and general open-mindedness. As employers we need to reflect the communities we serve and in the last ten years we have come a long way to achieving this. We have made huge progress over the decade but there is a lot more that can be done and bringing this back to Roland, developing ideas and innovation space and conversations for people to notice and act upon their own self-limiting beliefs and truths are essentials. If individuals are not receptive to the things they need to do to lean into their career, then all efforts are wasted.

LIVING DAY TO DAY

Sooner or later, you'll need to face the fact that you're living with this thing day in, day out. Some days you never think a thing about it. Other days it hits you like a boot in the face. You'll be on a bus and suddenly you'll think, 'Am I the only person on this bus to be going through this? Am I the only one with HIV?' Well, if you're somewhere rural and remote you might be justified for following that train of thought but if you're in London or one of the other big cities, chances are you're not alone!

As I've mentioned over and again, the situation for people diagnosed with HIV today is nowhere near as serious as it was twenty or more years ago. The older generation of survivors are sometimes vexed by the newly diagnosed person's attitude that 'It's only one pill a day,' but these days the medication prescribed is often as simple as that. The new mantra seems to be that if you keep yourself reasonably healthy and make sure you take your tablet every day, what can possibly go wrong? And, of course, if you suspect you've been infected and you get a move on, there is PEP (Post-Exposure Prophylaxis, a month-long course of HIV drugs that you can take very soon after sex which had a risk of HIV transmission, and can prevent HIV infection after the virus has entered a person's body). So what are we all flapping about?

Of course, it's not as easy as that. The psychological impact of the diagnosis aside, there are practicalities to deal with in terms of your physical health, not least of which is adherence to the medication – even if it IS 'just one pill a day'.

ADHERENCE – STICK AT IT!

You might remember from my story that at the beginning of my treatment I was taking thirty tablets three times a day. The times these were taken were highly regulated and I thank my lucky stars I had Richard to help me organise this into something approaching a coherent routine, using wristwatches and pill-boxes. Otherwise, I'm almost sure I'd have messed up and missed doses, leading to all sorts of complications. The side effects were bad enough; I certainly didn't need any adherence-related difficulties on top of all that.

While the number of tablets a newly diagnosed person has to take has dropped dramatically over a decade, you still have to adhere to regular days and times. You're likely to be told that 97% adherence is the standard, which gives you leeway of one missed dose a month. If you are less adherent your body starts building up a resistance to the medication, to the point where it becomes ineffective. So you've got, got, got to keep taking it and the very notion of doing that every day, for the rest of your life, can be scary. In effect, you're chained to this stuff forever and that can be a troubling notion.

Certainly, there can be mental resistance to the idea of adherence. Gradually you realise that you need to re-calibrate your life to accommodate a drugs regime and for some people this can be challenging. I remember taking one tablet that made me incredibly dizzy. I used to take it before bedtime so that I would be asleep during its worst effects, but Richard literally had to push me up the stairs. It gave me vivid nightmares and sometimes I'd wake up screaming. Come the morning I'd be fine, but dreaded the evening when it would all start again. Now I take my tablet just after break-fast, otherwise I feel somewhat nauseous if I don't eat beforehand. Other people might have to take them in the evening, so if you're out and about in pubs or clubs are you going to make sure you re-member at some point in the evening that your tablet is due? And if you take them out with you, how do you know that some bouncer won't stop and search you, then demand to know what your tablets are for? And if you're in company, or on a date, do you knock back your tablet at the table and leave everyone wondering, or do you pop off to the loo discretely?

Choices, choices; choices that make you a creature of habit against your will. And people don't like that, so they resist, con-sciously or not. My advice would be to swallow this –literally! If you weigh up the benefits against the inconvenience, there really is no argument. Whatever drug you're on, and however inconvenient it may be to take it every day, do remember that it's working to pre-serve your life. Granted, a young person's lifestyle is inevitably going to be more chaotic than the one I lead (!) but getting into the little habit of medication at regular times is a good one. It's about think-ing ahead. For example, I always carry with me a small docket of meds in case I guess stuck somewhere, and I can't get home. When flying overseas I always carry my medication in my hand luggage so as not to lose it, in the prescribed bottles and with the letter from the hospital saying that I must not be separated from my medication. It's a nuisance thinking that way, but the long-term benefits outweigh the grumbles.

THE FEAR FACTOR

...I was in complete shock when I was diagnosed, like everyone is. I just felt that there was a sheet of glass between me and the rest of the world, between me and 'normal' people, and I could never go back through it. I remember once driving up to the therapist's and behind me as I was parking was this whole family getting out of a campervan, and they were all laughing and chattering. I felt I could never be where they were ever again...

RUTH

I just remember darkness overcoming my brain, it just being black and I couldn't see any light. I wanted the world to swallow me up. I had a million and one questions, I was panicking, I was hyperventilating; I actually got quite angry and tried to throw stuff at the guy. I was just so erratic. All of a sudden, I felt in so much pain. If you've ever been in love and you've had your heart broken, it's that kind of suffering. You instantly want to be swallowed up whole by the universe, and to kind of disappear.

CHRIS

I have made logical decisions in my own head about taking my own life at some point. Especially if I'm in lots of pain and invisible and alone. That's not uncommon among older people anyway. It's not uncommon certainly among people who have illnesses, especially stigmatised ones.

DANNY

It brought it all back to me when I saw *The Epidemic* the other day. The memories were in my mind but when I saw all those emaciated people in the hospital, the cameras flashing around, and Princess Diana going to see them I thought, 'Gosh, don't ever feel that you are a bore because you still feel passionately about this'.

KEVIN

Something needed to change, so I quit my job. Having found just how much I valued my mental health, having lost it for a portion of the year before, I couldn't do that again. By that point I had already started my medication and that was going OK. For the next year I was living with friends, trying to find a job. I came out through social media, as HIV positive, on 2 October 2014. I felt that by being open and honest, instead of living in fear of my HIV, I could actually use this to own it and educate others.

JAMES

People are really shocked because I don't look unwell. I tell them the story of my bad experiences and my positive experiences and I finish it by saying, 'Have a test done, do it regularly, use condoms because of all the STIs', and then I also educate them about how you can't pass it on if you're undetectable, and that is interesting as well, they're like 'Ooh, we didn't know that'. I'm really happy to do Positive Voices, because I think I'm making a big difference in the community. The more schools we go to, the younger we tell them, the better.

FLORENCE

I keep promising myself that I won't dip into my interviewees' words (which you will read in full in Part Three of this book) but they're so good and so powerful that I just had to harness the above paragraphs. As Chris says, there is fear surrounding HIV – real fear. Fear of death, fear of chronic illness, fear of others' reactions and fear of an uncertain future. Fear that grips you in the night and refuses to let you sleep; fear that stalks you during the day and casts a shadow over everything you do and say. In many ways, and especially now, the fear of fear can actually outweigh the consequences of the illness itself. It is known that every year, three-quarters of people living with HIV experience depression, or ongoing emotional distress (ref: Positively UK, 'States of Mind' report, September 2013) and nearly two-thirds of those living with HIV live with at least one other long-term condition such as depression, hypertension, hepatitis B and C, cancer and diabetes (ref: Positive Voices, Public Health England 2015).

For me, the early period of diagnosis was terrifying. No other word can describe it. It was terrifying to the point that I wanted to end my life because the future looked so unpleasant. And I know I'm far from being the only one to have suicidal thoughts. There is no time limit on fear, especially if you allow it to dominate your life. And fighting it is exhausting.

I used to get up early, sit on the sofa and cry. Richard would find me sobbing over all of those panicky thoughts: 'What will happen now?' 'How did I get here?' 'What did I do?' 'Why me?' You feel so isolated because of that, and you believe no one else has gone through what you're going through. Looking back, I realise I'm incredibly lucky that Richard was there; for people going through this alone it must be a hundred times more difficult.

Fear never quite goes away. Kevin has lived with HIV for many years and has more than come to terms with his diagnosis but just seeing that documentary on TV brought bad memories and feelings flooding back. However, the good news is that it does subside after a while and your situation has become the new 'normal'. You might feel very 'different' to everyone else, but there again how do you know what everyone else is going through or feeling? Granted, they may be feeling healthier and happier than you – but possibly they might not. Being quoted the 'well, it could be worse' comment is a bit glib and not always helpful but if you really look at all your circumstances it's likely to have more than a grain of truth.

Dealing with the low times is all about calibrating them against the good times. For me, the positives in my life included having a partner who was still committed to me, having employment (though it was tenuous) and having a nice house to live in. Eventually, the ability to use my arms and legs properly and to be able to speak coherently came into the equation. Walking to the end of the road, slowly, became a thing to celebrate, as did the reduction in my viral load. It is important to celebrate small achievements like this, because it's about recognising and acknowledging the good stuff. And I can't stress too much how lucky I am to have had good stuff. I count my blessings every day.

Yes, of course I felt angry. Who wouldn't? It's normal, to be expected, because this is an area where strong emotions are easily unleashed. For me, it probably lasted for a year. The turning point came when I went as a delegate to a THT newly diagnosed course and through recognising emotions understood that the two biggest emotions I'd been feeling were anger and regret – and that neither were particularly helpful. Both use up a great deal of energy, and why not use that energy to do something more constructive?

For me, fighting the fear also involved a lot of taking ownership of the situation, as it were. I concur wholly with James when he says that being open and honest about his HIV status, instead of hiding in fear, means he can own it and help others. Whoever we are in life, and whatever we do, there is always an element of fear about the future – because inevitably, the future spells death. One way or another it will get me, and you too. So am I scared about my future health? No more than I am about getting run over by a bus, or being vaporised in a nuclear war. My only concern is that when my number's up, it isn't protracted, painful or undignified. And that's when the tablets come out...

This last point is controversial, of course. Others may or may not agree with this stance – that's a matter for them. Everyone has their personal philosophy and having the right to end my life when I choose to end it is mine. And yes, it brings me comfort knowing that I have settled this issue in my head – even if I'm far from crossing that bridge yet!

Do I think about my status now? Nowhere near as much as I did. It's just another fact of life, and there was no magic date when I realised I was no longer panicking about it. By degrees it subsides; it's an incremental thing. I do know that I started to feel I was rebuilding my life when I became a diversity officer and when I was running newly diagnosed groups. Those two elements gave me a sense of empowerment and fulfilment, and I think all of that came together at the same time. Today, having HIV makes me feel unique and special. And yes, different. Vive la difference!

PART THREE

WIDER RIPPLES

Welcome to Part Three of this book. This section comprises the narratives of thirteen individuals currently living with HIV. I reached out to the HIV community to ask for people who would be willing to share their account. Here are those that volunteered. The majority of them are white gay men, some of whom are long-term survivors. Others have been diagnosed relatively recently. There are three women; one white and older, the other two black and younger. Some have agreed to let me use their real names, others not. This is not a judgement on any of these great people, but a reflection on the stigma that still surrounds the condition so that some fear the impact that knowledge of their status could have on themselves or on those they care about.

While there may appear to be a bias towards gay men, it is the case that most people living with HIV whom I've met on newly diagnosed courses and long-term survivors' groups are just that. Had I had the time and space to widen the representation in this section, I would have done so. However, I had neither. That said, I talk to people living with HIV from many different walks of life all the time and I hope that what they share with me will one day be seen in print or online.

The narratives showcased here are arranged in chronological

order (year of diagnosis) in order to highlight how progress has (or has not) been made in areas of HIV/AIDS prevention, treatment and support over the last thirty years. They cover the full gamut of emotions from despair, anger, fear and isolation to acceptance, understanding and, in many cases, ownership of HIV. There are stories of medical and public ignorance and misunderstanding, particularly in the early 80s period, and new-to-the-market drugs which caused almost as much pain and suffering as the HIV itself. Through our narrators, we see how HIV can control every aspect of one's life (if it is allowed to do so) and how such a diagnosis can be interpreted as a force for good.

Courage is a theme that runs through each account. Courage in facing up to physical and mental distress. Courage in 'carrying on', even against seemingly overwhelming odds. Courage to stand up to loneliness and isolation, and courage to hold on to a future which sees the individual accept their status while not allowing it to 'become' them.

I hope you find these chronicles interesting, at the very least. They don't always make for comfortable reading, but where HIV is concerned there are few fairy-tale endings. That said, their unremitting truthfulness more than makes up for any lack of Hollywood schmaltz. Welcome to the reality of living with HIV in the twenty-first century.

At a service I announced that we were doing fundraisers for people living with HIV 'like myself.' Father Brian gasped and nearly had a heart attack...

NAME: MAURICE GREENHAM
AGE: 76
DATE OF DIAGNOSIS: 1984

Music and drama have always been an important part of my life, and have helped me through some difficult times. I came from a poor working-class family in Blackburn, Lancashire, but we had a piano. My dad started to teach me. He couldn't play it properly, yet he got pleasure out of it. It was there all my childhood. It didn't stay in tune very long, but the music I heard inspired me to become a member of the choir at All Saints church nearby.

I did well at school, though I failed my eleven-plus, and everyone was surprised at that because I was one of the brightest kids. I'd had time off for an injury – I broke my leg playing football, so I never played football again after that. But I did really well in secondary school and got eight O Levels without any problem. There was talk of me going to the local grammar school to do A Levels but my parents said, "No, he's got to go to work and support the family."

My first job was at a solicitor's, but I didn't like it and eventually got a job with the Ministry of Labour, as it was called then, at an employment exchange in Blackburn. I earned good money but when my sister went to work I decided to go to college in Durham and study to become a teacher. My subject was music and drama. My first school was a probationary year in Nottingham, with an awful headmaster. I got through that, then I moved to Macclesfield where I was in charge of music. After that I was poached by a girls' school and they said I could have a head of department post. This all happened before I moved to the Stoke-on-Trent area, where I am now.

I had a kind of mid-life crisis, which was about me coming out as gay, and in 1982 I left teaching. I'd always wanted to work in theatre and various people said, "Well now's your chance." I wrote 200 letters to all kinds of theatre companies and got 200 rejections, until I had an interview for an assistant stage manager's job at the New Vic theatre in Hartshill, Stoke-on-Trent.

I was offered the job and was delighted. A new career and a new life beckoned. Then, in 1984, I was diagnosed with HIV. I'd come back from a holiday in the United States with my partner at the time. We'd acquired a sexually transmitted disease, and we'd gone to a clinic in Atlanta, Georgia, for penicillin shots and for my partner it hadn't quite cleared up. So we both went to the local GUM clinic in Hartshill and unknown to either of us we were tested for this new strange virus that was causing AIDS. My test came back positive and his was negative.

I thought that somehow it had piggybacked on with the gonorrhoea. But of course, it doesn't work like that – you can't catch HIV from someone who doesn't have it. I was imagining this piggyback scenario and I know now it was just a load of rubbish. I was just making it up for myself.

Then I realised that three months earlier in Easter break, we'd gone across to Amsterdam, and I had had unprotected sex there. Shortly after that I had a bad flu-like infection, and didn't know what it was. My cure for any illness at that time was to go running and I ran the marathon in June, just before getting on the plane to go to America. At that time, I was actually HIV positive.

It was the head of department at the clinic who came and gave me the news. He was a lovely guy. We just sort of chatted and then he said, "Oh, you're positive to HTLV-3." He didn't really mention what the consequences might be. So, when I came home it just struck me and I thought, 'That's it, that's the end'.

I was totally devastated and angry too, because having just started working in the theatre as well, I thought I was going to lose all that. I thought, 'Who do I tell?' So I told those people who needed to know; my best mate, my best friends and my brother and sister. Not my mum – my dad had died by that time and she was getting on, she had enough to worry about. I thought I'd keep it from her.

I felt fit, and I thought, 'I'll just keep myself as well as I can'. I threw myself into my job because I was just at the start of a career that I loved. Anyway, from my first job I went on to Derby Playhouse as deputy stage manager and from there I went to Birmingham Rep and eventually to the West End.

I even acted! At one particular theatre they'd used up the entire budget on the stars and they had still to cast a character. I said, 'Look, I'll do it'. It was certainly not a big part – it was a butler – but it was an important part because he appears in every scene in the play. The read-through went perfectly well, and I got a good review in The Independent. That put the cat among the pigeons! So the director said, 'Right, you're in the next show'. I played Merriman in 'The Importance of Being Ernest'. I'd always loved acting, but I had the good sense when I was making the career decision to do stage management. Even so, I enjoyed performing and I've been on television as a supporting artist in loads of things.

I was offered AZT when it first became available, but I said very firmly, "No." The thing was that I was well then and working in a job that I loved. If I had been ill I'm quite sure my reaction would have been difficult, but I was well. I was informed, I'd been proactive about my health for quite a while. There was a very good Body Positive network and I was a member, so I got regular information from them. The general consensus was 'Don't touch AZT' as it seemed to be killing as many people as it was saving. If you were desperate you went onto AZT but if you were not desperate then you steered clear of it.

Then, when it was discovered that halving the dose was twice as effective, I still said, "No" because I was still in the same situation. It wasn't worth it, I didn't think at that point. Then in 1993 I realised things were not right – I was having memory problems and skin problems too; molluscums and warts and all this kind of stuff, and of course my CD4 count was going down rapidly.

The memory problems escalated from small things like losing glasses and keys to bigger items…like cars! I even resorted to having a tracker device fitted to the car, so when I would forget where it was I could go to the police. It was that serious. When it happened, I went to the police and said, "I've lost my car can you track it?" They said, "No way! We only do that if it gets stolen." So the next time I lost it I rang up and said, "My car's been stolen." That didn't work out either because I was phoning from a service station on the M6. At that time, service stations on either side of the motorway were identical. And I phoned up and they knew that I was probably phoning up from the wrong side. They said, "Can you go over to the other side and just have a look there?" And that's where it was.

The next big thing was when I lost the money to pay the actors. Fortunately, I went back to the digs I was staying in, pulled back the curtains and there was my briefcase. It was done in time, but I always knew when it was happening that it was not good.

So at that point I said, "Yes, I'll go on to AZT." I went on AZT for a few months, and then I was put on the first combination therapy that was possible in this country, which was AZT plus DDI. It was the delta-trial showing that the two drugs taken in combination were far more effective than the drugs taken separately. I gained time from that, but it was not nice to take because DDI are big, chalky tablets and must be taken on an empty stomach.

In 1994 my HIV developed into AIDS. My defining illness was encephalopathy, which was explained to me as early-age dementia. I was given six months to live. I thought, 'I'm not going to take that, in any way'. I thought that the thing that I needed to do was to keep my brain active, so that's when I started going back to education.

Having got through a year without dying, I decided in 1995 that I wanted to raise awareness and funds for various HIV organisations. I did this for a while but in a few years I was burned out. I was diagnosed with clinical depression, but I'd lasted long enough to benefit from, and suffer from, the new drugs. During this time I came out to the congregation of my local church. At a service I announced that we were doing fundraisers for people living with HIV "like myself." Father Brian gasped and nearly had a heart attack because he knew there were homophobic people in his congregation; in fact the overwhelming majority of people were wonderful, and that's applied every time I've been open about my status, especially to church congregations.

In 2004, I thought, 'I'm 20 years living with HIV – I've got to do something special'. I saw *Lord of the Rings* with all those amazing locations and I decided to take a trip to New Zealand. A former boyfriend was then living in Auckland and I thought, 'Here's a chance to meet up'. It was really good, I got on with him and his new boyfriend and their furry family.

For five years I went back every year, exploring more and more of the country. The year 2009 marked my jubilee, twenty-five years living with HIV. Again, I thought I should do something special... So that year as well as a trip to New Zealand I went to volunteer in South Africa with Hands at Work, a charity that looks after AIDS-orphans and does home-based care for people living with HIV. I went there as an openly gay man living with HIV, which seemed to present a problem for them. I said, "Do you want me to go home?" and they said, "No, we'll have to pray" and I replied, "OK, fine. I'll stay."

I got along fabulously with everybody apart from one or two of the volunteers. I went to White River, which is where the community was, and also across the mountains to Swaziland. It was a great experience, the people that I engaged with seemed to enjoy it and appreciated my being there.

I've now been living with HIV for thirty-three years and I'm 76 years old. I've got two honours degrees, both obtained after my AIDS diagnosis. I have also passed all the ABRSM organ exams including Grade 8 with merit. My confidence and self-esteem have consequently grown immeasurably. Of course, I'd like to do a Masters and a PhD, but I've got too many other commitments.

I get inspiration from younger people too. Last year BBC Midlands Today came to my house, to film a short piece with me and a younger person, fairly recently diagnosed. So, they had the two of us together as a comparison and that was really good because I was able to say, "Look, you might find this a bit of a surprise, but quite frankly HIV is not much of an issue for me anymore. I take my medication, and it's just once a day and that's really brilliant, the issues I face now are the health concerns of ageing just like everybody else."

Recently diagnosed people are not always younger people. At the National Long-Term Survivors Group, we introduced a weekend for recently diagnosed people. These have been amazing because, not only have younger newly diagnosed people attended, but also older people come who have been late-diagnosed and have ill-health in all kinds of ways. In both cases all you can do is tell your story and understand that you can live a really full life, to a normal life expectancy just like everybody else.

I really think that you must have a positive outlook on life. Funnily enough, I said I get caught up in all sorts of things, well, one of the groups I love being involved with is the Ages and Stages

Theatre Company, and guess where it's based? At the New Vic theatre. So I'm still part of the New Vic family after all these years.

And it's wonderful, absolutely wonderful. The thing is you get roped in to doing amazing things; the most recent was a conference on medical humanities at Keele University. It was a three-day conference and a group of us from the Ages and Stages Theatre Company attended. We did a workshop with all sorts of people – doctors, professors and people from academia; it's great, you can share ideas regardless of your background. One presentation introduced us to the concept of 'New Ageing', with a book that they recommended – I went off and bought it and read it in a day.

In the same workshop a couple of academics were looking at role-play with older people for positive identity. One of these was superheroes. They'd got pictures of older people in superhero outfits. Lee, a professor from Plymouth University, pulled out an old shirt from his bag and slung it around his shoulders like a cape and said, "When was the last time you threw a cape on your shoulders?" and I said, "Last Saturday" because I'd organised myself a gold cape for the parade at Stoke Pride. Lee was impressed.

So what are my future goals? I would like to obtain a diploma for organ playing to up my game another notch. The same goes for academic studies. I feel I could get a Masters and then a PhD. I'd really like to do that because people I've encountered who have done a doctorate seem to have a better grasp of knowledge and to be more articulate than people who haven't. Then of course I want to continue globetrotting. The last two years I've realised that I was passing over countries to get to Australia and New Zealand and then going all the way back over them again. I thought, 'Why don't I break the journey up?' So last year for the first time I bought a round the world ticket. I went to Thailand, Singapore then to Australia and finally Indonesia. This year I went to Vietnam, Australia and New Zealand.

When I arrived home this year, Father Brian said, "Oh, thank goodness you're back in time for Candle Mass." What he failed to mention was the guest choir he had invited. That's the sort of situation I come back to. No matter, I find music a great source of consolation and inspiration…as indeed is being part of a community. It's good to have people constantly around you, always looking out for you. Joining groups takes up time, but it's worth it: people look after you, they inquire after you if you're not there, and they ring up to see if you're alright. I always make time for people…for me it is vitally important. In my book you should always find time for people. If there's no time…you just make it, that's the way life works – well that's the way it works for me, anyway.

The doctor who was overseeing my blood tests said to me, 'Well, you're gay, you probably have AIDS, so we're going to test you for it'.

NAME: DANNY WEST
AGE: 57
DATE OF DIAGNOSIS: 1985

I'm a working-class boy. I was born and grew up in North London. When I was a kid I wanted to go into acting but I did one play with the BBC and hated the whole experience. Then at fourteen I became a volunteer for people with learning disabilities and enjoyed that much more.

I left home when I was fifteen because I was beginning to identify as a gay man at that stage and my family's attitudes were not conducive to a comfortable home environment. It was pretty scary. I felt excluded from family life, and I continue to do so to this day.

I could barely read or write when I left school. I was dyslexic, which of course in those days wasn't called dyslexia: it was defined as being stupid. Even so, I signed up for a residential childcare course at the City and East London College. Then I got my first job as a basic grade residential social worker when I was seventeen, and spent about eight years working in residential care with people with learning difficulties.

I just threw myself into work and it was at that point I started to meet other people – gay men and women anyway. I remember marching on the Gay Pride event back in the 1980s where we supported the miners. I'm still friends with one of the guys who was one of the organisers of that event and was depicted in the *Pride* film. I became quite politically active with NALGO, which was a public-sector union. I got involved in some of the gay rights stuff going on, and that was the beginnings of my activism and equality and diversity work.

I started clubbing when I was seventeen or eighteen and built my own circle of gay friends, engaging with the gay community at The Black Cap in Camden and places like that. Then I started doing my social work qualification when I was about twenty-two, which I obtained a couple of years later. Then I became a manager of a residential home.

In 1985, when I was twenty-four, I went for a regular sexual health screening appointment. The doctor who was overseeing my blood tests said to me, "Well, you're gay, you probably have AIDS, so we're going to test you for it." At that point I had only just started to hear about the 'gay plague' or whatever they called it then. I'd only just started reading stuff about it in *Gay Times* and I didn't know much about it. But it was pretty scary, and I hadn't considered for one moment that it would be something that would or could affect me.

I was quite taken aback by this doctor's suggestion that I might have it. Anyway, they did the test, essentially without my consent, and said come back later. So, I went back to my small group of friends in the horrible damp flat we were living in and told a couple of them that I'd been tested. One of them was a bit shocked; nobody really knew what to say or do. A friend of mine agreed to come back with me to get the test results. So we went back, and the doctor said, "We've tested you, it's positive and you've probably got a year to eighteen months to live. We suggest you get your affairs in order." And that was what amounted to post-test counselling.

I didn't expect that result. It shocked me. I was completely immobilised by fear, it was like, "How do I deal with this? Oh my god I'm going to die." We left the hospital, went back to my flat and we all were in complete shock. Nobody knew what to say or do, so we opened a couple of bottles of gin that night.

Quite soon after my diagnosis, my parents started the process of divorcing. I confirmed with them that a) I was gay, and b) that I had HIV. And my father said he never wanted to see me again or speak to me again and he never did. He died about five years ago.

Then I went onto AZT and then DDI. I had so many side effects – vomiting, acute diarrhoea, seizures, skin problems, all sorts of stuff. Within six months of going on those I decided that I wasn't going to carry on the treatment. Actually what I wanted was quality of life rather than quantity. If I was going to spend the rest of my life feeling like this, I might as well come off them and deal with it. Friends rallied round and we all tried to get information. A particular friend found out about an organisation called Body Positive. They'd just started to have pub nights at the Market Tavern and she dragged me along kicking and screaming really. I found myself in a pub with about twenty or thirty other guys. All of them had also been diagnosed; some were healthy, some were clearly very sick and some were clearly dying.

I was sitting at the side with my 'girlfriend', my female friend, on my own. I had to try to go over and talk to people, I was terrified. Eventually I did spot a guy at the bar whose name was Graham Gardner. A few days later I met him at Hammersmith Broadway tube station, and we became lovers. He had a diagnosis of AIDS at that time. He then suggested that I come along to a meeting with him to meet a guy called Christopher Spence. I went along to this meeting of gay men and we talked about an idea of setting up a centre and a hospice for people living with HIV and people with AIDS. So that's where the idea of the London Lighthouse started.

I became part of that initial group and we started running workshops mostly for gay men in those days. They aimed to empower people, to enable people to think about death and dying, to be part of a peer network, all that kind of thing. I became close friends with Christopher Spence, and that community developed quite quickly with all sorts of people. Then over a couple of years, London Lighthouse was built. I was involved in that community for many years, meeting lots of people and making lots of friends, most of whom are dead now. I watched lots of my friends die. It was a very traumatic time. A very painful time.

Graham died about four years after I met him. We were just friends by then, but I was at his house when he died and I remember the undertakers taking his body away in a black bag which had a special zip on it, which meant you couldn't open the bag. So I wasn't even able to say goodbye to him. That memory has always stayed with me and it was that then that finally started me addressing my grief. His death, the loss of the people around me and the potential loss of my own life.

Soon after I was appointed as the first local government principal training officer for HIV and AIDS, located in Hammersmith and Fulham. The social services in that borough were the first local authority to have referrals for people with HIV and AIDS, and quite significant numbers of them. There were all sorts of problems and all sorts of reactions from staff across the board within the local authority – dustbin men refusing to take the rubbish away, things like that.

Later, all other local authorities looked to Hammersmith and Fulham to help them develop policies and address services and figure out strategies for the challenges HIV/AIDS presented to local authorities. I ended up travelling all over the country delivering training. We worked incredibly long hours, and there were all sorts of very distressing incidents, and very stressed people who were in terrible circumstances, many of whom were dying and did die.

I stayed at Hammersmith and Fulham for a few years, then I met my first long-term partner, Nick, who was much younger than me. He was from an upper-middle class background and he wasn't positive. It was pretty much at that point that I decided to leave the HIV sector. Nick said, "Come on, we've got a life to live", and we went off and bought a house in the country.

I lived the life of Riley for a while. We travelled, did whatever, spent ridiculous amounts of money. When I met Nick, he wasn't out as a gay man. He hadn't told anybody in his family, so when the relationship progressed in the early years, we went through the process of him coming out, which was tricky. I met the family and then we explained to them that I was HIV positive. They welcomed me with open arms and I became very close to them. I became a bit closer to my mother at that point, because I was spoiling her rotten.

The thing about HIV, which I have learnt over the years, is that it's just a virus. That's all it is. Viruses have killed large numbers of human beings and they always will. And somebody always gets blamed. If you look at the history of any disease, there's always one society or community that gets blamed. HIV raises all the issues that society doesn't deal with very well. When you talk to someone about HIV, it presses all their buttons, if you like. You think about sex, you think about death, you think about illness, you think about addiction, you think about racism, you think about all the things that you don't talk about. If you tell someone you have HIV, you're also asking them to think about all those other issues, and the majority of people just shut down.

When I think about my father's reaction, what I know about my father is that all those issues are ones he couldn't handle or deal with. So I'm not particularly surprised now that he reacted in the way that he did. And I guess that enabled me to come to terms with his reaction, though it hasn't made it any less painful. What I wanted him to do was embrace me and reassure me, and he wasn't able to do that.

In the early 90s I remember taking my mother to one of Lighthouse's workshops. We had a residential workshop weekend for people with HIV and their parents. She found the whole experience very distressing. She just couldn't handle the emotional side of it. It was very terrifying and very traumatising in some ways for her. She stayed for the weekend and then she said to me, "Don't ever do that to me again." It was her telling me that she didn't want to talk about it, and she's continued not to talk about it.

I don't think I've had a conversation with any of my brothers about being gay or about HIV. They've always excluded me from family life. I get the occasional invite to things but nobody talks about it or me or what I'm doing. I'd like to know the strange ideas they have about the sort of life I have. When I am with them it's very isolating because I can't talk about my life, I can't talk about who I am, what I am or what I do. So, it's just, "Hello, how are you?" then I'm stood there on the end, not feeling involved or that I can contribute in any way.

One of the things I remember thinking when I was hanging out in the hospital when I was diagnosed, was that I'm not going to die of AIDS. That there were too many things I needed to do in life. I've always been very goal driven. I always knew that I wanted to travel. I was the first person in my family to ever go to college. I was the first person to ever come out as gay. Once I got into the Lighthouse community, I was very clear that I wanted to be part of the human rights debate around people with HIV. After Nick and I split up, I came back to London. I was unemployed, homeless and had no money. Eventually I got rehoused. So, I've always lived in social housing and I was never in a position to buy my own home, and I'm still not in that position.

Now I've set myself up as a learning and development consultant within the public sector, working with disability and HIV. I've done a lot of work with the Terrence Higgins Trust, and a lot of the HIV organisations that are around at the moment. I just continue to work in that field and I've always enjoyed it.

Healthwise, there were moments when I thought I was going to get an AIDS diagnosis (but never did), and times when I was actually quite sick. I ended up being a patient at the Thomas Macaulay ward at the Chelsea and Westminster. I was a patient at London Lighthouse on a number of occasions. I went back on medication while I was with Nick, and eventually found the regime that worked for me and that had minimal side effects, and continued to have treatment ever since. I'm now undetectable. I just take three pills a day, every day, and that's it. I've moved from seeing my doctor every month, to seeing my consultant every nine months. If there are any problems then I go back and see them.

I guess the most current issue for me is about growing older with HIV. Firstly, I never expected to grow old. I certainly haven't made any provision for it. I've never had enough money to get a pension or a house and I still live in social housing. So a) I have lots of concerns about that and the future, and b) I never psychologically thought about or strategised about getting old, and what that would mean to me physically.

I don't have family around me and although I have friends, as you go through life you lose them and as you get older you have fewer friends. I don't really have a picture of what being old might be like, though sometimes I get a glimpse of it. I live on my own, in an isolated part of London. I don't know anybody locally. I don't have any support networks locally. I don't know my neighbours. I'm in a community where I have no friends, nobody I know at all. It's a nice quiet flat, and it's affordable, which was one of the reasons for moving in the first place. But I am very isolated. I have visions of me being sat on my own as I get older and older and older and I've got this spinal problem, and when I go into spasm, I can't do anything. No shopping, and I can't even get in the bath. I've found myself in situations where I've been completely alone here and it's like, "What the hell do I do?"

I have made logical decisions in my own head about taking my own life at some point. Especially if I'm in lots of pain and invisible and alone. That's not uncommon among older people anyway. It's not uncommon among people who have illnesses, especially stigmatised ones.

As a long-term survivor now, I tell the younger generation my story so they can begin to understand and comprehend what it was like in the 80s. That's why it's important that books like this are going to be written and the documentaries that I'm in are being made. I think we do need to chronicle that story, we need to make sure that story is not lost, that it's told. So I find myself engaging in conversations where I'm giving people accurate information, and I guess I'm challenging people. Not in a negative way, but I'm encouraging people to explore their own behaviour and what the implications of that are.

What is different now is the message I tell people today isn't, "Hello, I'm Danny and I've got HIV." The message is "Hello, I'm Danny and I'm undetectable." That's a huge difference. That's actually very empowering, to be able to say that. People ask, "What does that mean?", and I can say that I tested positive, however I am now undetectable and can no longer pass on the virus. That's a very different opener if you like. Yeah, I think I've started to get slightly different reactions.

What would I still like to achieve in life? Well, I've recently started working for a project organising events and provide befriending and information to the older LGBT community. I've started to find myself becoming part of the older LGBT community, and actually when I talk about HIV in that, it's very well received. They're very supportive. I guess I will become an old man, an old gay man, and will become part of that community. There are things out there for the older LGBT community, social opportunities and stuff.

I see that I will get more and more involved in that as I get older. I've been working on an empowerment model, called 'The Social Model of HIV', which is a model that perceives HIV as an opportunity to develop and hone a whole range of skills. I've been developing that for the past couple of years for people with HIV. One of my goals at the moment is to continue promoting developing that model, and start to put together some empowerment programmes for people with HIV. So I'm sort of still working on that.

I don't really have a life plan, I'm just taking it day by day at the moment. I carry on doing the work that I do. I try to make sure that I don't get isolated, by staying in contact with friends. If you're heterosexual and you've got family, it's different. If you're gay, you often don't have family, or you may have been rejected by your family because of your HIV status. So you have to work at it a little bit harder. As long as you're around people who embrace you and accept you and all that. I'm very clear that I've contributed an awful lot over the years, I'm very proud of that. So, in that sense it's been a life worth living, because I have influenced events and had an impact on people's lives. That's why I continue to do the work I do.

There were things in the newspapers saying to round everybody (with HIV) up and put them in the old TB hospitals. There was another thing saying, 'Gas them all'.

NAME: CHRIS
AGE: 54
DATE OF DIAGNOSIS: 12 SEPTEMBER 1985

I've had an eventful life, but what have I done? Nothing significant really. I often have this feeling that people I know who have died would have used the time much better than me. They would've done more with it, or had more fun or whatever. I think that's the most disappointing thing, and maybe that's why I wanted to be an architect, to sort of leave some kind of monument.

I'm from Greenwich, London. Basic working class. I went to a secondary modern church school in 1975 and then that was it. I wanted to be an architect. I always had a thing about nice big buildings because I grew up on a council estate. But it wasn't really encouraged at school. I had a career day and I remember the headmistress, she was just like Mrs Thatcher. She came up to me and said, "And what would you like to be?" and I remember saying, "I'd like to be an architect" and she looked me up and down and laughed and said, "People like you don't become architects."

After school, I went into nursing. I did my general training, but I started off in psychiatric nursing because we weren't really in a position for me to go off to university, so I had to get a job.

I never came out officially. It was more sort of a situation that was forced on me because I had my partner, and I suppose from that it was obvious. Then later on he died from AIDS, and up until that I think everybody was in denial, nobody spoke about it.

We were both diagnosed in 1985 and he died in 1988. How

long he'd been positive before that, nobody can really know because the test didn't exist. He came home one day and sort of said, "Sit down" and I sat down on the bed and he said that he had been to the clinic and he had found out. He said that he had spoken to the health adviser, and that she had said that it would be a good idea if I came in and got tested.

So that's why I went. And yeah, it was a shock. In those days there was nothing, no treatment. I had the test and then of course I had to wait the three weeks for the result. The health adviser said to me, "You're positive for HTLV-3" (which was how they described it then) and I said, "Well, what does that mean?" and she said, "You'll be dead within three years."

There was nothing else to offer. She said, "All I can suggest is that you try and live as healthily as possible. Try and avoid being around other gay people." Nobody knew anything about the routes of contamination or anything. They were just clutching at straws. I had been there because of my partner and she had seen him and thought because he was messing around all the time, that I would be doing the same thing. I wasn't, I was just sitting at home being the faithful partner and had all this thrown onto me.

I must've gone into shock because for years afterwards, I always thought the date of my diagnosis was 5 October 1985. Much later on I asked the clinic to check the date for me and it was the 12 September. So I think I must've just closed down for three weeks. I didn't dare tell anyone. There wasn't anybody you could talk to because there was all the panic in the press, everybody was getting sort of psychotic about the thing, and then there were all those terrible AIDS adverts. There were things in the newspapers saying to round everybody up and put them in the old TB hospitals. There was another thing saying, 'Gas them all'.

We were absolutely terrified, the two of us. Something would come up on television, or in the papers and we would just sit there and look at each other, we wouldn't say anything. It was terrifying.

I told one friend, Michelle. She was a nurse; I felt safe telling her. But I couldn't tell anybody else, and then there was the added problem that I was in nursing. People were saying that healthcare workers who had HTLV-3 should be withdrawn from work. A while afterwards, when I went into general nursing, I was forced into a position where I had to tell somebody and that was really scary. The problem was, being in general nursing, I would have to work with children. That meant that I had to be immunised for rubella. So I approached one of the tutors in the school of nursing who was quite obviously gay. I went to see him, and I said, "I've got this" and he said, "Listen, I don't have the answer, whether it's safe or not." He said, "I'll do is some phoning around." Eventually he came back and told me it would be OK. He said, "Don't worry, obviously I'll keep this under my hat." So I carried on working as much as I could.

The diagnosis affected me more mentally than physically. I've only realised years and years after to what extent it affected me. I have obsessions now with things like death and dying. When you're told you're going to be dead within three years, then obviously as soon as you're told that you're waiting for it. Then you see your friends die around you. Then your partner dies. Then you get to those three years and you think, 'Any minute now...'

Every single year you get an illness and you think, 'Oh God, this is it'. I've had some bad illnesses. I had cancer; lymphoma. That's actually an AIDS-defining diagnosis. That was in 2000, so officially I've had HIV since 1985 but I've had AIDS since 2000. I've had pneumonia a couple of times as well. Every single time I'm thinking, 'Oh God, I'm not going to come through this'.

I've always hoped, not just with the HIV but when I had the cancer as well, that I would have some kind of revelation or epiphany or something. I've always sort of hoped that that would happen, but it didn't. It wasn't like suddenly I learnt that I've got to grasp life – I've just sort of stumbled through the whole thing really.

For the first eight years I never did anything. I was in complete denial. I never went back to the clinic for a check-up or anything. I was preoccupied with my partner because he was dying and that was a long process. I was still partly nursing him at home, then he actually chose to go in to hospital.

He was sent to the Middlesex Hospital, which I think was the first AIDS unit that was opened. That was difficult, because I was doing my training, so I was studying and working. Then, because we were living in Brighton I was driving up and down to London for the hospital. I was doing that five times a week. It was just exhausting, and then there was all the stress when you went in to the ward. In that ward I remember seeing the impact of AIDS on the other patients. The people covered in the Kaposi's sarcoma. I remember seeing a guy who had gone blind from it, and another young guy who had senile dementia. People seem to forget now. They think that AIDS just sort of manifests itself in one way – that you just get thin, and you die, but it doesn't, it's not one illness, it's a syndrome of illnesses and it can manifest itself in a hundred different ways. I was not only seeing my partner, I was seeing my own future in each of these guys and thinking, 'Well, which one is going to be me?'

From the mid '90s I started going to the clinic because I'd started to get sexually active again. But, I didn't even want to talk about HIV to the doctor, you know, it was just for other things. When I had the lymphoma, I was living in France then, with my present partner, Claude. I had been having incredible pain and the STI clinic referred me to a psychologist because they thought the pain was stress-related. He told me I was having panic attacks. I told him "I don't feel panicky, I'm panicking after I get the pain, not before I get it" but his reply was "I know what I'm talking about, I'm the clinical psychologist. You don't know, just listen to me and do what I say." I went to see a cancer specialist in France and he said to me "I don't know what it is you've got, but I can guarantee to you that it isn't cancer" and he referred me to the clinic for tropical diseases as he thought I had some kind of tropical disease which hadn't yet been discovered. I eventually saw another cancer specialist who, after MRIs and scans, diagnosed me with a huge tumour on my spine and I was sent to the institute in Marseilles. They were the ones that started me on HIV medication. I said, "But I don't want to go on medication" and the doctor said, "You've got no choice, because you have a viral load now." She said it would just be stupid not to take medication.

I had the chemotherapy, which lasted months. Then after they had finished that, I had to go in to hospital to be operated on to have what was left of the lymphoma removed. I had to have a cage put on my spine.

To consolidate it, I had to have a bone graft taken from my leg to put into my spine. Then I had to be operated on again because they needed to tighten up the cage. Then once all that was done – that took several weeks – I had to start radiotherapy. Oh, I had the lot, and then there's the rehabilitation because I could barely walk afterwards. So, I had a lot of physiotherapy, about 200 sessions. This is why I'm constantly obsessed with death and dying all the time. Whenever I get a pain now I'm thinking, "That's it, the cancer's come back." It's like my partner said; he's not the most sympathetic of guys, but I guess what he said is true. He just said to me, "Let's face it, what choice have you got?" You've just got to get on with it.

I had a bad experience at A&E in France a couple of years back. I had been having chest pains. I was put in a bay (one of several all in earshot) and the nurse started taking bloods. After a while she came back with my hospital notes looking furious. "You're HIV positive!" she said out aloud. "Why didn't you tell me? Are you trying to kill me?" I stayed calm and said I hadn't said because it's already on my notes. She hadn't used gloves and came back with "You could have ruined my life." I stayed calm and said, "Working in A&E you should assume that everyone is HIV positive. You don't know if an unconscious person is negative and lots of people don't know their status. Until you know for sure you should automatically assume that a person might be positive; that's the protocol in most countries." She shouted "Well it isn't here!" There were people in the other bays listening and I said, "You don't know about any of these people. Even if they say they are negative it doesn't mean they are." I saw a little boy and said (obviously not loudly), "How do you know that little boy hasn't got HIV?" To which she (as a qualified nurse!) replied, "Because it's a child, not a gay man." The consultant heard the noise she was making and came out to ask what was happening. The nurse told him her view and I added "You should assume everyone could be positive unless you know otherwise" to which he, as a casualty consultant replied, "That's stupid. That's like saying that all drivers are potential killers." I replied, "They are!!" To think this was just a couple of years ago. It's shocking that in a modern western country health care professionals are still so ignorant.

I was with a woman for a while and I've got a daughter. This is nothing short of a miracle really. Not the fact that I did that, but the fact that she's not HIV positive. It's a long story and I was very open and honest about my status (and the fact I'm gay!) but the woman wanted a child and that happened. I haven't been allowed to see my daughter since she was eleven, nine years ago. People say, "She'll probably come looking for you when she's older and has children of her own", but I think how much longer am I going to be around for? Just before I met her mother I'd been in a relationship with a skinhead lad whose friends had no idea he was gay. Eventually they did find out and subsequently he fell to his death from a tower block. I do wonder whether it was an accident or not… I couldn't even go to his funeral because his mother didn't know anything about his sexuality.

So much had gone on in my life that some years ago I considered ending it. It was a culmination of years of denial mixed with years of just waiting for HIV to hit like some grim reaper following me around; constant memories of my two partners who had died, the friends lost to illness and the dreadful things I saw in those early days on the AIDS ward of the Middlesex hospital. I had other problems going on too like the long running problems with my ex in order to see my daughter, a family who wanted nothing to do with me and there was also the fear of the cancer coming back which still haunts me now. I was drained.

I was sitting at home one evening with my partner watching TV. He said, "What's wrong with you?" I didn't know what he was talking about and he pointed out that I had tears flowing down my face. I didn't feel like I was crying but I was. I just said, "I don't know."

At some stage before that I had contacted someone and the plan was to meet the following night when my partner would be at work. I had no previous knowledge of this person and had contacted him through some dubious website. This person agreed, for a fee, to inject me with something that would end my life. It was part "I can't go on with this anymore, just waiting" and part "This is the only way I can take control…get it before it gets me" that drove me. I felt absolutely nothing while arranging it. No emotion. I was like a robot.

The day following that evening in front of the TV, I sent a message to the guy to confirm. Evening came and I waited for my partner to go to work. I just said "Bye", like I always do, and then calmly showered. I got into the car and drove to the address I had been given which was about an hour and a half away. The address was some village. I can't even remember the name now. I found a car park, parked and set off to look for the place. I remember it was an old village house. The door was on the street and the guy came to answer. He took me up some stairs to a kitchen. He explained that he would give the injection but I would have to touch the syringe to make it look like I had done it myself. I just said "OK". I handed him the money. We sat at a table and he started preparing things. I just watched. As far as I can remember I wasn't thinking about anything. I don't know what the product was. He apologised for preparing in front of me but said he didn't want to get it prepared beforehand in case I didn't show up. He said he was ready and I offered my arm. He stuck the needle in and moved it around a bit, pushing it slightly this way and that before saying "I can't get a vein, let's try the other arm." I gave him the other arm without a word. He tried again but still could not find a vein. He said, "You've got no veins!" I didn't answer. I don't think it surprised me because I always have problems for blood tests etc. He went back to the first arm and tried for a third time. No luck. On to the second arm again for a fourth try pushing it this way and that. But nothing. He pulled out. He was going to try a fifth time but at the same time said that he didn't want to just inject anywhere because he couldn't guarantee the result. He wanted to be sure of a vein for a quick result. At this point it was as though I woke up. Suddenly my head started working again and I was more aware of where I was. I just thought, 'There's a reason why he can't get a vein, I'm not meant to do this'. I stood up and said, "Forget it." I apologised for wasting his time and told him to keep the money. I drove home and just went to bed as if I had just had a normal night.

I don't talk about HIV much now. I keep myself to myself really.

The only positives really that have come out of this is, the partner that I'm with, I've been with longer than anyone, we've been together eighteen years. That helps a lot, because you're not constantly faced with the question of having to tell a potential partner, you know. We did it once, and I've not had to do it for eighteen years. When you meet a new partner, you have that dilemma a lot.

I haven't really been very ambitious since I got diagnosed, I've basically just been cruising through life. Scratching my way through and just making do, you know? With everything else it's, 'What's the point? I'm not going to be around to see it through, if I do this or the other, you know. I could die'. People say to me, "Well, you could die anyway, you could be hit by a bus." If I hear that sentence one more time, yes, I could be, but that's something that's out of the blue. I know I have HIV-AIDS, so that increases my chances of something happening tomorrow. So I've just sort of been strolling along, falling all over the place and into things. A hundred people can tell you to grab life by the horns but it makes no difference: it either comes from you or it doesn't. Life's not all about winning, sometimes it's about just being.

On one HIV site, someone said to me from Africa, 'I think you boys tell such wonderful fantasy stories, if you've been living with HIV that long that's impossible'.

NAME: KEVIN KELLAND
AGE: 66
DATE OF DIAGNOSIS: 5 DECEMBER 1986

I was born in Gibraltar. My father was in the Navy. Both parents originated from Devon; Newton Abbott and Paignton. My father unfortunately caught polio in Gibraltar and had to be flown home. I was a babe in arms at the time. Dad was at Stoke Mandeville Hospital being nursed and unfortunately, he never walked again. But he returned to work for the Admiralty as a writer, and then mum and dad saved up for a bungalow in Plymstock near Plymouth and returned to their roots. That's where I was brought up. I would say it was rather middle class, back where I came from. I had a brother as well who was younger.

I always knew in the bottom of my mind that I was gay. I had lots of girlfriends, and I liked women very much and I think I was in love with some of them, but there was something that wasn't quite right. I came out in about 1974, when I was twenty-three. I remember I saw the film *Cabaret*. I was at the cinema with my brother and his now-wife, and a girlfriend. I thought, 'Oh my gosh, that's me, living this double life'.

Gradually I dipped my feet into the water of going into the gay bars and it was quite scary at first. This was a very secretive world that was accepting, that you felt like you belonged to. I never told my parents at the time, I was always a bit scared. I spoke to my father later on. My mother always came over as rather anti-gay, saying, 'It makes me feel sick' and all this, you know? Those one-liners that people say. My mother unfortunately died in January 1994 of cancer. It wasn't long after my HIV diagnosis so in a way I was glad I never told her, because I might have blamed myself. It was hard keeping things together with her going in and out of hospital. She was very establishment my mother. I loved her to bits – and I think this was very much the right thing to do. Her death was devastating and I suffered stress for a year afterwards.

In 1985 I had a relationship with an Italian man, he was lovely and I really fell madly in love with him. Then towards the autumn of '85 I had a letter to say he was HIV positive. I had a couple of tests, which were clear, then in 1986 I met a gay doctor and went out with him. I thought, 'I'll be safe with him'. I didn't use condoms, I did not listen and by November '86 I thought, 'I've got a feeling about this'.

I was decorating at home – the spare room – because my Nan was coming to stay for Christmas. I was listening to a radio programme and I thought, 'I'll just get that HIV test again'. So, I went along and they said, "Oh, you look fit" and so I had the test. Then they rang me up and said, "Well, we want to check again."

They told me I was HIV positive on 5 December 1986. Lovely Christmas present, wasn't it? I was very shocked. I remember I didn't sleep at night. I used to turn off the TV when all the HIV stuff came on. I was very scared.

I had a full-time job as a photographer in one of the big stores there, and on the day I was diagnosed I was so numb I just walked around Plymouth and I thought, 'What am I going to do with it? I just don't know what to do or where to go'. So I went to work and I told two people – one lady was about forty-five and the girl I worked with, Tracey, was eighteen. They knew that I was down, they knew that it wasn't just that I was fed-up with work, and so I told them. They were upset but took it in their stride. I remember the frightening thing was that the next day Tracey was late for work and I thought, 'Oh my gosh, that didn't go quite as well as I'd hoped'. But she came in late because she'd only missed her bus – to my relief.

Thankfully that was it, and they stood by me. All those years I worked there, they kept it confidential, it was our secret and they were there to support me. I'd taken the risk, and I could've been sacked, you know what people are like, 'You can't take our portrait, you can't come near our toddlers and babies, posing them in groups'. I took that big jump very quickly and survived it, and I got my confidence, and I decided that I was not going to tell my parents until I became ill. That was it, I thought, 'There's no need to tell them'.

There were plenty of support groups, I must say that. There was the Plymouth support group and I was offered help, but I didn't want to go to an HIV support group. Instead I was offered help from an Anglican vicar because I was a liberal Christian, and he gave me quite good support. Then I got involved with Plymouth Body Positive, run by a Roman Catholic priest, Father Ronnie, who was a fantastically down-to-earth guy. He was so supportive and said, "Why don't you use your sexuality and status as a gift? I'm sure you'll go far with those in need." They were very good, some of them. They just got on with it. I trained as a buddy and I went from being numb to an 'AIDS Crusader'.

I wanted to know more about HIV and I started working alongside the health advisers in Plymouth. I worked side by side with them and I felt it was just a place where I found myself. I didn't actually get interviewed, I just grew into it; today in fact I've outlived some of them – the health advisors who helped me in the beginning. That's rather sad.

Some of my friends I actually had to buddy. I remember one was a bit reluctant, and said he didn't need help. I remember going in to see him and he was delirious, he was so ill. I remember coming out of that visit with the two health advisers and we were crying in the lift of the hospital. There was my friend Anthony who I had met about a year or so after my diagnosis. He was the dashing blond type of man and we were friendly for a while. He came from London and had family in Cornwall.

Then one day he walked in to my studio and he looked very ill. I said, "Oh, hello, you don't look too well" and he said, "No, it's the big one, I've come home to tell my family. I've got AIDS, I'm on my way" and I said, "Let's have a cup of coffee and talk about it." I remember he stayed the night at my place. I took him back to Cornwall and he wouldn't let me drop him at his parents' place, I had to drop him around the corner. I left him and he just walked away to his parents' house. I didn't hear anything more from him, and then Terry Roberts who was the health adviser said, "Do you think you can help this man we've got? He's having trouble with his family, they're evangelical Christians, they're Methodists. He's at the Royal Naval Hospital. Can you go to him?" When he said the name I thought, 'It's Anthony'.

I started visiting him in the Royal Naval Hospital, every day I used to go after work. His parents were lovely, but sort of a little bit misunderstood the whole situation. One of his sisters was an evangelical Christian and she said, "To save his life he has to be cast out of devils." I remember seeing Anthony that evening and he said, "Am I damned now?" He would always put his thin hand on my face. When I went to the hospital I always thought, 'Am I going to find the bed stripped and he's gone?' but in the end, he was moved to a respite home, which really was for elderly people. That's all they had in those days. He died in September 1989. It was a particularly moving experience, being with him.

I've always been a very liberal Christian. There were plenty who wanted to give help, they weren't all 'Wrath of God', they just wanted to get on and help. So I was in Jersey and I met this very dashing Irish guy called Brendan, who was an ex-monk. We got talking, and he'd lost a friend with AIDS. I always remember he said, "Look, we'll keep in touch." We kept writing and he eventually rang me very excited and said, "Look, I've been working with some Roman Catholic nuns who do AIDS support work in London. We're setting up this place for people with HIV/AIDS called Bethany in Cornwall." I started going to the meetings in Bodmin with the health advisers, nuns, and a collection of this, that and the other. Gradually we fundraised for us to open the old children's home, which was opposite, and until then we had five or six people who could live, or have little holidays, in the annex.

That was a wonderful time of spirituality and deep camaraderie. We raised loads of money, we sent letters all over the world to institutes or businesses. I used to have cheese and wine parties which would raise £500, in my little two-up two-down. It was a marvellous project and we refurbished the place, it was like a hotel. Princess Diana came and opened it. Bethany served people with HIV till about 2003/2004, but I left the project around 1995. Then Brendan left as my father was on his own then and I couldn't really give him much time. I got involved in the Devon AIDS Association, I was always involved in something. But it was a wonderful place that served people for a good thirteen or fifteen years.

Ironically, my health was generally good. I had terrible IBS around '95, nearly nine years after the diagnosis. It was the stress of losing so many people, and also my mother had died. In 2001 I had pneumonia and they thought I had pneumocystis carinii. After being ping-ponged from my GP to the hospital, I was admitted to hospital on the fourth time, they put me in a wheelchair and took me right up the ward and admitted me immediately. Then they said that I didn't have pneumocystis, I did have pneumonia but it wasn't pneumocystis. But I felt very, very ill. It took me about three months. I remember it was my fiftieth birthday in the September. I got myself fit enough for that and I took my first trip to San Francisco.

In 2004 I had two heart attacks and was very ill from those. I survived but unfortunately caught giardia, which gave me terrible stomach problems, and diarrhoea, which made me lose a lot of weight, which was after the operation. One friend of mine said, "You look just like Freddie Mercury." However, I wasn't put on HIV meds until 2006. They said that my CD4 was too high. I think I was down as a 'non-progressor'. They put me on Sustiva and I was a bit nervous of taking the drugs because I'd seen what the side effects were, although I knew they were saving people's lives. I was hallucinating all night and I remember that I went to the bathroom in the morning and stood up to urinate, came out of the bathroom and collapsed. My partner Steve had to ring A&E. Eventually I went in to hospital to see the HIV-consultant and they changed those tablets immediately. From there on they put me on Kivexa, and then they said that after a while there was heart trouble related to that, and since I'd already had it, we don't want that. So, now I'm on Truvada and Rilpivirine and really, they're just like taking vitamins, there's no real side effect. I'm one of the lucky ones that really swam through the rough water and came out the other side.

That said, it was difficult, very difficult, being HIV in the early days. All you wanted to be was around people who were HIV-positive or under the umbrella of HIV. You didn't want people to know, you didn't feel like you were in the dating game. I remember I did eventually go out and date people, with my condoms, and practised safer sex. But if I was going to go into a longer term relationship, I'd tell them, you know. A couple of partners I had, they'd never let on, but they were a bit frightened.

I met Steve, my civil partner now of twelve years, on 1 January 2005 at a club in Torquay. It was about a week after we met that I told him. He was quite shocked but his brother, who's also gay, had an HIV-positive partner, they got their heads together and said, "Yes, you can do dah, dah, dah," all this, so really it was – unbeknown to me – a good support.

We married, or had a civil partnership, in 2011 when I was sixty. That's the time that I decided that I wanted to do all the things that I never could've done or was too scared to do, because now I'm sixty I can! I went to a Mary Wilson (of the Supremes) concert, who I've been a great fan of. She said, "Would anybody like to come out on stage and sing with me?" I went up for it and we all sang with her, I never believed that I would have the courage to do that.

I think a lot of people, maybe rightly or wrongly, hide their diagnosis and they could do a lot more good with it. They're so scared of mucking up their lives, and then you might go and say to someone, 'dah, dah, dah' and you find that they've had graffiti and dog's mess in the door. You just don't know how it's going to go. I remember once I put one line on Facebook about being HIV, I said "Oh yes, I've been HIV-positive but it was then twenty-seven years ago" or something. It was a one-line remark but Steve said, "You don't know who will see that, I would delete it immediately" which I did. Then I was going to do a talk for the Red Cross about living with HIV. So, I thought, 'I'll put that on Facebook'. It was sort of 'the launch' of coming out. Then on Facebook people were saying, 'Oh I didn't know' and all this. I don't think one person said anything disrespectful at all. On one HIV site, someone said to me from Africa, "I think you boys tell such wonderful fantasy stories, if you've been living with HIV that long that's impossible." But, I think that's the only thing I ever got.

Most people said, "You're very brave, it takes so much courage to do that." I remember when I came out, I did some television on World AIDS Day, and I also was in the paper telling my story. I was out walking the dog and people were like, "Oh, you're the man in the paper, fantastic story, I was very moved." All similar things like that. I think it needed someone who was just ordinary to say it.

When I talk to younger people, I notice they seem to think in the back of their minds, 'There are tablets now aren't there?' I know some people with and without HIV who take tremendous chances. I mean, now that we have PREP I'm reading that there are other strains of things like gonorrhoea that they can't cure. But it's good to see younger people doing some activism. They take on board what we went through going forward into this new era now.

We worked so hard, I think it brought it all back to me when I saw *The Epidemic* the other day. The memories were in my mind but when I saw all those emaciated people in the hospital, the cameras flashing around, and Princess Diana going to see them I thought, 'Gosh, don't ever feel that you are a bore because you still feel passionately about this'.

I've got friends of mine, they've done their bit and they don't want to know anymore. They don't like my things on Facebook, they stay clear of them. I mean, they're friendly in other ways, but they're just indifferent. I think I just want to leave a legacy of my life and the history of HIV in Devon and Cornwall, which I put, a face to it. Leaving a face to that era can't be forgotten. I mean, that's my achievement, I would like to really leave that history. A legacy of my life and the other people who either died of HIV or helped with HIV. I'm proud to do that, and passionately want to do it, very much.

When I talk to younger people now who say, 'Oh, HIV is just about having one pill' and all that I want to do is slap them silly. Because it isn't just a pill. They're still writing the textbook.

NAME: STEVE CRAFTMAN
AGE: 60
DATE OF DIAGNOSIS: JANUARY 1987

If I were to rate my quality of life now, out of 10, I'd have to put it at 2.5. I've got more T-cells than I had, and an undetectable viral load. It's just the drugs that are trying to kill me. I've had a variety of illnesses and I can't walk without a stick. I live in a small village and if I need to go anywhere I take a taxi. I tend to try and keep things upbeat. I live alone. I can walk as far as the village shop and even that walk is slow and painful. In two years I've had perhaps four, five people who weren't Sainsbury's deliveries guys come through the front door and I spend 99% of my time alone. I don't know any other gay men, apart from online. So, as a person who has lived with HIV for more than thirty years, my message to younger people is – 'You don't need this'.

I was brought up in the North East of England and I came out in 1976 when I was nineteen and at university in Birmingham. Really, I should've been in care in the 1960s. I had parents who were self-involved and emotionally manipulative. It was psychological bullying, basically.

I got involved in gay politics in Birmingham. I realised that I shouldn't be at university. I'd only gone because it was what the family thought I ought to do. But I took a coldly cynical look at a student grant compared to what I'd get on the dole and stayed at university for the rest of the year.

I was working as a volunteer at the Peace Centre on the promise of a job when turnover increased. Then I moved down to London, when my then-partner got a job, and basically we opened a squat.

I was very quickly involved with Gay Switchboard and when I broke up with my partner I moved in with the 'Brixton Fairies' (legendary London gay community of the 1970s). It was when I was living in Fairyland that I think I seroconverted. What happened was that my housemate came home from the clinic in a stinking temper because he had got secondary syphilis. We both had identical rashes. So I went to the clinic expecting to be told I had secondary syphilis. And I was told, 'No, we don't know what this is, but we've been seeing a lot of it recently, so have some calamine lotion'. That was my first HIV medication. One thing that wasn't known about at the time was seroconversion illness, so I thought nothing of the rash I'd had.

At the time I was doing knitwear design and production knitting, so that was basically what fed me, but my real interest was in working at Switchboard, which led on to working at the National AIDS Helpline.

In 1986 somebody I'd had a fling with died. My thought at the time was, 'If I didn't have it before, I've got it now'. We knew the chances of transmission, but it took me till the beginning of 1987 to go and have the test. It was a three-week wait then. The day before my three weeks were up I phoned the clinic from the Switchboard office to ask if the result was back.

The way the health advisor said, "Yes, I do have a result for you" I thought – it's positive. I said, "You're not going to tell me over the phone, are you?" She said, "You know I can't." So I went from Kings Cross to Balham and got the positive result. "Yeah," I said, "I thought so," and went straight over to Acton to go and do a shift on the National AIDS Helpline.

For the first twenty-four hours it was, 'I know something different about me'. I knew something new about myself. I was thirty, and my first thought on diagnosis was, 'Well, at least I don't have to worry about having a forties crisis'. I didn't fall apart until the next night, when I was talking to a friend I knew was positive and that's when I lost it. He looked after me, took me home with him and made sure I was alright. I worried a lot about it over the next couple of months and then thought, 'Hang on, if it's a really valuable secret, what's the best way of making it worthless?' And the answer was to make it freely available, so I've been out since then.

At the time it was all, 'Poor you, tragic person you,' but in all fairness there was no treatment and so many people were dying, it wasn't unreasonable. The first however-many times, you accepted the sympathy, but you end up hearing how brave you are too many times and eventually I got pissed off hearing that and thought, 'Let's fucking do something about this'.

The first TV I did was 1988, with Miriam Stoppard. It was all, 'You have the virus which means you're an AIDS carrier' and at that point I remembered a piece of advice I had been given a while ago, which was, 'Anytime you're being interviewed on TV and they say something and you want to stop, you swear'. I looked her in the eye and said, "I'm not a fucking AIDS carrier."

They stopped and said, "Well, what do you want to be called then?" And I said, "I'm HIV antibody positive", which was the way we were phrasing it at the time. My then-boyfriend's ex, who subsequently became my partner, looked very much like me and he got followed around Woolies by a bunch of kids asking if he was on TV the other night. The only consequence I had was that I was teaching a couple of adult classes in machine knitting and I lost a couple of students. I'd warned the college that I was going to be on TV and what I was going to be saying, and I expected that to be taken into consideration if my class numbers suddenly reduced. I was basically saying, "Try to end my courses because of low numbers and I will see that as discrimination."

I ended up working in Westminster city council's specialist HIV homecare team. We were the second one in the country – Kensington and Chelsea got there first. I lasted about two years in that job, because I knew I was slowing down. The last six months I was in the job I ended up doing the more social worker end of the job, rather than frantically vacuuming and cleaning.

Then I moved to a social work team, and by that time Stuart and I had got together. Stuart had gone to Australia because his mother was dying. She died about a week after he got there. We had to sort out her house and I had a phone call from him, "She's just died, how soon can you fly out here?" I said, "Next Tuesday?"

Stuart was ill with HIV when we were in Sydney. We got back to the UK in the middle of winter and he went pretty much straight in to hospital. He wanted to buy a house with the money his mother had left him, and I had the job of viewing properties. The one he actually bought was one we viewed together, and he got to live there for a few months before he died. His will had been written with the expectation of what my life expectancy was likely to be, and it was considered to be eighteen months. And here I am, twenty-five years later.

I got on to do AZT via the concord trial. My doctors placed me on to the low dosed arm. I got my AIDS diagnosis through untreatable herpes and although I stayed at sort of arc levels I had many chest infections towards the end of the '90s including one AIDS-defining one and the most appalling skin condition that they never identified. I was itching so badly that I tore myself to shreds. It was so bad that you could see the pattern where I'd been sunburnt several years before. The last AIDS-defining illness I had was cryptosporidiosis in 2008.

I was on a Nevirapine trial in about '96. I can't remember but it was the only way you could get 3TC. Which is why I went on the trial. That lasted two years and they rewrote the trial protocols, after the first year to allow the unstructured protease inhibitors. I went from about eighty to about 250 CD4, in that time. So I got halfway towards recovery.

I'd met a guy within six months of Stuart's death. John got sick in 2003. He'd tested negative several years on the trot and stopped testing because the way he liked sex there was no HIV transmission. But he worked with homeless men and one day in 1998 he had been first on the scene when somebody had been shooting-up and they'd hit an artery. He got a face-full of blood. He had a dose of shingles in 2000 which worried me a bit but I shrugged it off with 'He's in his forties – it's when people start to get shingles…' But then he also had a needle-stick injury at work in 2003. By then they'd got the HIV rules sorted out and he'd had an immediate HIV and Hep-B test. HIV came back positive, and on further investigation he had just eighty T-cells.

He was sick with MAI, it took him two months in hospital to find that out, but he survived longer than anybody else I've known with MAI. I nursed him for the four years he was sick. By the time that we moved from Bristol, John was very obviously ill. I'd been through the twenty-eight inch waist jeans that kept slipping off phase and I think I went down to about eight-and-a-half or nine stone through malabsorption.

After John's death I started rebuilding life. In 2011 I felt I'd regained enough health to get a motorbike again. I'd stopped biking in '96 on the grounds that, 'I can't do this anymore, I'm going to kill somebody'. So I got the bike and totalled it. It was the night after a storm; I was on the worst bend between the village where I lived and the nearest shop, which was nine miles away.

I ran over a branch which was rotten, lost balance went over and broke my ankle. Around that time, the woman who had been my best friend in the village suggested that I move down south to where I am now, just outside Neath, West Glamorgan. So, I gave up the council tenancy to move here. I was very sick when I moved here and was getting sicker. I ended up being told, "We want you in hospital on Tuesday." I couldn't figure out why it was that, in four days' time.

It turns out it was time to draw up the papers to have me sectioned. I had Fanconi syndrome caused by Tenofovir. It tends to be slow onset.

The hospital I had been going to hadn't been monitoring my blood properly. Or hadn't known how to interpret the results. I had dangerously low potassium levels. I was hallucinating all over the place. I don't really remember 2012.

Now I get standard rate care and advanced rate mobility. I had to appeal to get the enhanced mobility – basically, I can't walk without a cane. HIV-wise I'm fine. I've been on eighteen different drug combinations and I'm on Darunavir with Cobicistat because it's cheaper than Ritonavir.

I'm a member of a number of groups on Facebook. I just stepped down as the moderator of a kink board in America because my libido finally gave up the ghost a couple of years ago. I'm more bothered about the fact that I'm not bothered about sex!

So this is just my normal, and when I talk to younger people now who say, "Oh, HIV is just about having one pill" and all that I want to do is slap them silly. Because it isn't just a pill. They're still writing the textbook. I believe that we don't have the science yet to produce a drug that's going to actually be a cure. We've only got holding action drugs. Who's to say how long they are going to last?

Basically, what I'm hearing is the immortality of youth. It's condom fatigue. They were only ever meant as an emergency measure because the whole mess would be cleared up in a few years. There still isn't a condom on the market that's been designed for anal sex.

The makers have had over thirty years to work out a standard, work out a design and they've not bothered, because nice people don't go putting willies up their bum. I do advise, but only insofar as you can on Facebook. I try to keep to the rules of speaking in I-statements, and all the rest of it, except when somebody comes out with something offensive, and then I open up with both barrels.

I expect my standard of living to go down, not up. Men in my family tend not to live out their sixties. I've got diabetes and am at high risk of heart disease. Diabetes was acquired through protease inhibitors. Basically, I expect to spend the next ten years coffin-dodging.

I knew in that moment exactly what had happened to me, I knew in that moment exactly what he had done to me.

ANDY
AGE: 43
DATE OF DIAGNOSIS: OCTOBER 1997

I was born in Liverpool and I grew up on The Wirral. I'm now forty-three. I've always known my sexuality, from when I was very young. I remember being about five or six and being in the garden with nature, and having a picture taken. You can see from that picture that there is a gentleness of my being, a softness of my masculinity.

I was sexually abused when I was twelve years old by a family member. I really wanted to experience the physical touch of a man. When my uncle came over to stay on holiday, Easter-time, another bed was set up and he stayed in my room. It was really very confusing for me, because, as I say, it was something that I sort of wanted to experience. The power of touch, and that male union, closeness, connection and bond. You're completely blinded by that when you're twelve years old, you think you know what you want.

When I went to bed that night I couldn't sleep, I was awake with my curious mind and thoughts. Even before he came in to the bedroom, it wasn't all that late, but I'd been awake because it was the holidays and you're allowed to stay up a bit later. I was pretending to be asleep, feeling fearful and panicky as much as excitement and wanting to be asleep, but the wanting to experience and the thinking had kept me awake: 'Is it going to happen now?'

He was joking and jovial all the time. I was very drawn to him in that respect. He made me feel very at ease. But I didn't realise the enormity of the psychological effect until all these years later.

I don't even know how I fell asleep. I must've been that tired, I finally went out in the small hours of the morning, I'm thinking about four or five, when I couldn't stay awake any more. I didn't want to make a big thing of it in the night and disrupt the whole of the house. I was scared and felt like I couldn't move couldn't move, lying still in the dark and in silence.

I thought I would wait until as soon as someone had woken up, my mother or father. Mainly my mother as I was close to her, I wasn't really close to my father. I was waiting to go to her. Anyway, the morning after I did, I broke down and shared it with her. She was consoling me, holding me.

I wasn't hugely successful in my GCSEs as a result. I did OK, considering what I'd been through. I excelled at the things that I enjoyed i.e. drama. I went to Butlins and worked for a while, to get away and to feel freedom within. Before I left for Butlins I told my parents I was gay and it was then I was told that my dad wasn't my real dad and as I'd not really had a father/son relationship it didn't come as a surprise. Whilst at Butlins I wore a red coat and people asked me if I was a redcoat, so it was entertaining to say I was when actually I wasn't, it was a lie, I just wore a red coat. I worked as a fair-ride operator.

Anyway, long story short, I got the sack from there, it was like a scene from *Prisoner: Cell Block H*. I was escorted to the gate with my belongings. Then I went to Blackpool, from there to Birmingham, Manchester and Liverpool. Ten years after I was sexually abused I was raped in Manchester and purposefully infected with HIV. I was training to be a croupier at that time as I saw that it was a chance to travel the world. I could go anywhere with this skill. The world was my oyster.

So I was based in Liverpool, living at my Nan's at the time, and I was training between Manchester and Liverpool. I got quite drunk one evening and I'd missed my last commute home to Liverpool. I was a little bit stranded, if I'm being particularly honest. I was in and around Manchester Piccadilly basin because there was a gay cruising area which I was familiar with and I thought maybe I might be able to meet somebody there, friend or foe, that might be able to put me up. It wasn't just for sex; it was more for a roof over my head if I'm being completely frank.

So, if I were to meet someone attractive, fantastic, that would be a bonus. My real need was for accommodation for the night. So I met this individual down there, I did recognise him, his face, although he was a stranger, we had never spoken, and he invited me back to his. We got a taxi back. He was older than me. I was twenty-two; he must've been around thirty-two. On the way back, we went via an off-licence and he said, "Oh, would you like to get some more vodka?"

I said, "Yeah, yeah, why not?" He was welcoming me into his home for the night, the least I could do was put my hand in my pocket and kindly offer him the money for the drink. When we got back shortly later he said his neighbour next door could get some cannabis and would I like some? I said, "Yeah" giving him more money again. I was out of it. I remember noticing packages of condoms about, the ones you pick up in gay bars, placed here and there. As soon as I'd seen them, it made me feel safe. Now looking back, I think and feel they were placed there strategically, to make me feel that way. Looking back on it I think that was a bit of a trick and part of his web of deceit.

Nothing sexual happened immediately when I got back that night. I collapsed on his bed and was out of it. I slept face down. When I woke up in the morning, I woke up to him having sex with me. I thought I was having a nightmare but in actual fact it was reality I had woken up to. My immediate thought was, 'Why would somebody want to have sex with somebody when they're asleep?' and, 'Has he got a condom on?' The first thing I said to him was, "Are you wearing a condom?"

Just in case he didn't hear me because I had just woken up and if I hadn't said it quite loud enough, I asked him again. And, I repeated it for a third time. His response was complete silence; that was his answer. He darted off to the bathroom and he insisted to walk me back to the city centre, as if nothing had taken place, like as if everything was just like it was before and nothing had happened or changed.

I lay frozen still when he went off to the bathroom I was still face down, hungover. I knew in that moment exactly what had happened to me, I knew in that moment exactly what he had done to me.

My world in that moment shattered into a thousand million pieces. My world literally spun around. I was disorientated and dazed. My life in that one moment had changed forever and I had no control over it. I was vulnerable. I had already been drinking when I met him. It was easy for him to do what he wanted to do to me. I was powerless.

I knew straight away, I knew in that moment. Why would a stranger want to have sex with another stranger when they're asleep? People would only do that if their intentions were something more disturbing. People don't do things while people are asleep unless they're doing things people don't want to know about. Simple. I am not stupid, I wasn't born yesterday. I knew in that moment exactly what he wanted to do, and what he'd been successful in doing.

I wanted to get away from him as quickly as possible. I wasn't immediately angry with him, I was more completely shocked – shell-shocked would be an understatement. The right things to do in that situation aren't the things that you necessarily do. You should do 'A', 'B' and 'C' but when you're a victim of that type of experience, 'A', 'B' and 'C' go right out the window, everything stops, pauses and runs in slow motion; you lose all sense of time. I think it was more survival really, trying to keep calm and under control. I was completely in shock, scared and fearful.

I went to Liverpool for an HIV test. I'd only been for a few tests before and they'd been negative. The result of this didn't surprise me. I told them what had happened to me, but the nurses couldn't even be bothered to write down the word 'rape'. No police were called to me, nobody was called to me, no support was given to me. What was given to me was, 'You're HIV positive, there's the door' end of story.

As soon as I got my result back, I wanted to go and see this individual again who thought he'd screwed my life up and threw it down the gutter with no conscience whatsoever. I was mesmerised, it's too much of a nice word to give to him but it's how I felt, about his behaviour. I went and faced him. I told him that he'd been the last person that I'd had a sex with and the positive result. He replied, "What are you trying to say?" I said, "Look I'm trying to say to you that you're the last person that I slept with, this is the result." He responded, "Oh well, I've got HIV positive friends who go around the gay village who have sex with young gay men to give them 'the gift'." That was his own confession to me, in that exchange.

I was ridiculed by him and his associates from then on. It wasn't until 2006 I went to the police. I wasn't going with any hope that anything would happen at all. I went there because I couldn't take any more psychological trauma. I got to a point where I just couldn't take any more. I was going there thinking that even if nothing happened, it might give him a scare, or if he'd done it to someone else, which I know 100% he must've done, that when the next person is brave and finds the courage to come forward about this individual, and I'd been the first, they would be treated better than I was. They would be more believed and supported.

After the investigation the police told me because I went back to his consensually as an adult, and that they couldn't prove the fact that I'd been raped because I'd gone back consensually they could take no further action. They also said that, "We're not supposed to tell you this, but you're doing a lot better than him and he's got cancer."

So, not only did I feel that I was let down by the police, and let down by the nurses, but I felt let down by everyone and there was nowhere I could talk. I went to George House Trust (a HIV support charity in Manchester), which was the only place for me to go to, they said, "Welcome to the HIV family."

Once, I went to a retreat for therapy and when I brought up the subject of the rape I was always told, "We'll come back to that." I was silenced, pushed aside and disregarded. My rape and HIV come part and parcel; they were asking me to split myself into two.

I've exhausted all the support from the friends I had. I've got plenty of friends around me but there are only so many times you can speak to the same friends about it. How many times can I burden my family and friends?

In 2009 an organisation called Survivors Manchester was set up, an organisation primarily to help men who've been sexually abused and raped. I had received support and psychological therapy there before. I reconnected with them because I found out they had a specific male therapy for sexual trauma. I went and did a four/five-month intensive talking therapy, through them, for men, because that was exactly what I felt I needed at that time.

Months later I was asked by Duncan at Survivors to become a member of an EAP (Expert Advisory Panel). He really values our input, because we're four different individuals with four different experiences that have been through the process. It's really helped me a huge amount. I shared at the meeting, "I'm really keen to do something as soon as the next thing comes up." We all are passionate about raising awareness for Survivors Manchester.

I said to Duncan, "Next time something comes up, bear me in mind." So anyway, about a week later he got an email from the Manchester International Festival, asking if there was anyone that was feeling comfortable enough to raise awareness for Survivors Manchester. He sent me an email and although it was quite daunting and scary for me, it had come at the right time. I used to use the word coincidences, and it's nothing to do with coincidences – its synchronicity. Everything happens at the right time if you are willing to make it happen and be aligned, and find the courage to push yourself through the difficult attachments and violations.

The universe is on your side, you've just got to allow yourself to be open. Put yourself in the right places and things will come to you. You've got to allow yourself to work at it and be in the right place with yourself in a non-judgemental, self-negative talking place; a heart-centred place.

I had been given an amazing opportunity; they placed a 100-metre yellow-brick-road catwalk through Piccadilly Gardens, and they shared my experience in four short pages. It said, 'Andy wants you to know that he was raped. He wants you to know that he was purposefully infected with HIV. Andy wants you to know that he went through hell, but with the help of Survivors Manchester, his Mum and Buster (my dog), he got through'. When I got to the catwalk the producer, Karen, said "When you get to the end, open your arms, open your wings, angel." So that's what I did when I got to the end of the catwalk.

I felt tears in my eyes; it wasn't tears of sadness. I felt a sense of relief; the applause and the love from the crowd. I felt like I'd scored a goal at Wembley. It was the rapture and the volume of the love that I could feel around me. The crowd was accepting me, it was overwhelming. It was really powerful for me, I'm really, really proud of myself. So many other new opportunities are opening up for me now. I've been asked to become a BBC Radio Five Live guest editor and there's a project called Islington Mill with three women in Salford who are designing wallpaper and putting it on exhibition in the

Northern Quarter. It's about my journey, darkness and finding my enlightenment. With this art you're encouraged to touch it, because when you touch it, it the paper opens up and you're be able to travel through my journey with words, dialogue and pictures.

Now that I'm opening up, nothing's holding me back any more. Standing on that catwalk was saying, 'You don't have any power or control over me. I take control and power back in my life.' I've got purpose and direction in my life now. I choose to go this way in my new life; I've been able to shed the old layers of myself, and I've found a piece of me that I'd forgotten about.

I've got direction and purpose, I've got love and light through the love of my brothers and sisters I now have in my life. I am happy every single day. Heaven is a place on earth. You've got to put the work in, you can't expect it to come knocking on your door. But I have been able to reach out for help and I choose to have the right people around me.

What hopes do I have for my future? The hope for my future would be that me speaking out and sharing would shine the light on the places that have really helped me out, so other men wouldn't suffer in silence as much as I have. That would be the hope. It would be for other men to allow themselves to reach out if and when they're ready to talk. To let them know about these places, because it's not about my experience, we've all got experiences. It's about them knowing about the places that can help them, that's all it's about, awareness. I hope that other men can be open to change, acceptance of themselves and the realisation that that they deserve love and can have a life of love again. We have all the answers and all the love inside of us. We may feel that places, organisations and even other people may help. Only we can truly make the changes, we have our own destiny in our own hands. The choice is ours to make and everything we will ever need is inside of us.

I told an ex-partner. He said, 'I'm going to have an HIV test and if it comes positive I'm going to find you and I'm going to shoot you dead'.

NAME: FLORENCE OBADEYI
AGE: 45
DATE OF DIAGNOSIS: 1999

I'm forty-five now and I was born in Nigeria. My father is Nigerian and my mum is Jamaican. My parents met in London when my dad came to study accountancy and my mum was studying nursing. They got married in Stoke Newington. Then they had my sister, and they lived there for six years, and then decided to migrate back to Nigeria. I grew up in a small town near to Lagos. I've got a brother, and a sister who's dead now, but there were three of us growing up.

When I was young my mother never talked about sex. I wish she had done. She was a very loving mum, and she took care of us very well, and I had a very happy childhood. That was the only one thing I wished that she talked to me about. The only way I learnt about sex was by reading books that were on the shelf. There was a book on biology. It had details about sex and pregnancy and things like that, but no sex education in terms of picking up infections.

When I went to university I had my first boyfriend and I was having unprotected sex. Then I started taking the pill. I was advised by my friends, "Just take the pill and you're fine." I was not thinking of sexual infections or STIs.

When I finished university, I taught in a secondary school as a general science teacher. I did that for a few years, and then I migrated to the UK. I met my ex-husband, who is also Nigerian. But that marriage did not last; he was seeing someone else and eventually I had to stop seeing him.

In 1999, I found that I was pregnant via an English friend I'd met. I went to the hospital to have the normal antenatal testing. The midwife suggested I have an HIV test. At that time they were testing women from certain parts of Africa – East Africa and South Africa – but not so much West Africa. So I said, "No, I'm fine, there's nothing wrong with me, I don't have HIV, I don't need to take a test," She said, "You can never tell, and also there's medication now for people living with HIV, to stop the baby from getting infected." When she said that, it made me remember the BBC news, where they were announcing the medication to save children from getting HIV. So, it clicked in my head and I thought, 'OK, I'll do it, I'll do it anyway'.

I did the test, and then I went home, and two weeks later I got a letter saying they needed me to come back to the hospital for further tests. I thought it was for diabetes or high blood pressure or anaemia or something. I went back to the hospital. A midwife came up to me and invited me into a room, and when I sat down she introduced me to a counsellor who said to me, "Your HIV test has come back positive." I immediately became distressed, I started to sweat, I was very shaky, crying; I became emotional.

It was a big shock, because I thought there was nothing wrong with me and felt fine. My understanding of HIV at that time was that once you're diagnosed with it, you're going to die. The counsellor spent one hour with me, talking about how HIV is passed on, and not to worry, I even said to them, "Could I have got it through care work – looking after the elderly?" They said, "No, you couldn't have got it through that. You can't pass it on that way. It's through unsafe sex, sharing needles and mother-to-child transmission." They kept on talking about the child, "we're going to do this to the child, the child will be fine", and then I said, "What about me? You're talking about the child, what is going to happen to me?"

They said, "There's new medication now, and the medication

seems to be working." So I felt a bit better towards the end of the counselling session. But then I went in to see a consultant, who said they had got the blood tests back and my viral load was in the thousands, very high, and my CD cell count was fifty. I don't know who infected me, because by the time I got diagnosed with fifty CD cell count, the doctors said they thought I'd had it for ten years before my diagnosis. I think I picked it up in Nigeria. I didn't bother myself about trying to figure out who it was.

Anyway, the consultant said, "You might not feel unwell, but in terms of HIV you are very unwell. Before the end of your pregnancy, if you don't take medication you will fall ill." I said, "OK, I will take medication straight away."

I took my medication, and then I summoned the courage to call Positively Women, and the woman I spoke to said, "Don't worry about it, I've been living with it for five years, I'm fine, just take your medication" and she invited me to the next group. I went and the women were all so nice, and I was surprised at what I saw, because I saw people with their nails done, make-up on, looking good. You could never tell anything was wrong with them. My impression of someone with HIV was someone who was frail or thin or you know, someone that's looking ill and unhappy. They were happy, they were full of life, some of them were pregnant, you know. So, that was my experience.

I felt a bit more confident. I was worrying – will this medication, work, and everything. So, when they told me, "Oh, I've been on medication for five years" or "I've been on medication for four years," it gave me confidence and motivation to want to carry on fighting, and make sure I take my medication and live.

I decided to tell the father of my child. He said, "OK, I'll go and have a test done." Two days later he came back and said his test had come back negative. Eventually when I had my baby, I rang him again to say, "The baby is here – come and have a relationship with your child." He started giving me excuses and saying he had children with three other women and he didn't really plan to have another child. He was concerned about the baby, he kept on saying, "Is it positive?" I said "No, he's not, he's been tested." At that time they used to do a test at six months and then eighteen months. All the tests came back negative and I told him. After I told him the last results, he changed all his numbers. I couldn't get in touch with him.

I also told an ex-partner. He said, "I'm going to have an HIV test and if it comes back positive I'm going to find you and I'm going to shoot you dead." That scared the living daylights out of me. He's someone I know, if he wanted to do that, he could. It was really scary, he went and did the test and the test came back negative. He never apologised for saying that to me.

And then I told a friend, he was just a friend, we didn't have a sexual relationship, just friendship. I'd known him from when I was back in Nigeria, he used to be our neighbour, so he knew the family and everything. I decided one day to tell him. He immediately got nasty and said, "Look at you, look at what you've done to yourself." He stopped calling me. That friendship just died there.

I had a baby boy. He's seventeen now. He's fit and healthy, yeah, he's fine. He's alright. The first five years, when I was living with HIV and bringing up my son, every time my son had a fever or anything I would panic. I kept on thinking, every time I took him to Accident and Emergency, I'd say, "Check him for HIV, check him for HIV."

When he was about five, I was watching a programme about a school in Uganda and they were talking to children as young as his age about HIV. So, I called him and said "Come, my son, and watch this" and we watched it together and he talked to me and said, "What is HIV?" and I said, "It's a bug that people get through having unprotected sex, sex without condoms."

I explained about sex, pregnancy, the dad and mum, the real story. I didn't make it up. I was preparing him so that when I told him about HIV, he would understand. I told him it's transmitted through sex and sharing needles and mother-to-child transmission, but the difference between the HIV bug is that people are scared of people that have it. So, they get treated badly, sometimes friends will become bullies or not very nice when they know.

A week or two weeks after, he saw me taking my medication, he's always seen me taking medication, and actually once I told him it was vitamin tablets. But then, as I was getting ready to take him to school, he saw me take a tablet and he said, "Mum! It's not vitamin tablets, is it?" so I said, "OK, remember that programme we saw on telly, about the people with the bug, HIV?" and he said, "Mum, have you got it?" He laughed, he thought it was funny.

So, I said to him, "Please don't tell them in the playground because it's Mum's private business and I don't want you sharing it in the playground because I don't want you to get bullied."

He was very understanding of that and some months after he came back and said, "Mum, do I have HIV?'" I said, "No, you don't have it, because I took medication," and then I said to him, "You know all those groups I go to? Well this person, that person and that person, they've got HIV as well. All the people you see when you go to play in your crèche, their mothers and dads have HIV."

He's been OK since then, and now if anything comes up with HIV, he comes and he tells me, if he sees it online or on the telly, he calls me and says, "Oh, come and see, Mum." And, that is when I try to talk to him about it, because he's a teenager now and he doesn't like to be bothered and he says, "Oh no Mum, I know, I know, I know."

My parents died before I was diagnosed and it took me two

years to tell my brother. He lives in Ireland, he's a pastor. When I told him, he just prayed for me. It's fine to pray for me, but show some emotional support by being in touch! He only calls me once a year. It's a cultural thing. When I was growing up in Nigeria, if we heard that someone is unwell there would be superstition around that person. My mum was not like that because she was Jamaican. She would go and see the person, support them if they had any needs, try to help them in the house. But Nigerians will avoid them, because they still believe in the devil or something. So there's superstition about illness: if you go around someone that's ill, you will get ill as well, or it will bring you bad luck.

Generally I've been in good health. In the beginning I had really bad side effects, I was really ill. I had very bad dizziness, heart palpitations, headaches, vomiting, diarrhoea. But nowadays, on the medication I'm on now, I'm fine. I volunteer for Positive Voices, going into schools and talking to community groups. People are really shocked because I don't look unwell. I tell them the story of my bad experiences and my positive experiences and I finish it by saying, "Have a test done, do it regularly, use condoms because of all the STIs." I also educate them about how you can't pass it on if you're undetectable, and that is interesting as well, they're like "Ooh, we didn't know that." I'm really happy to do Positive Voices, because I think I'm making a big difference in the community. The more schools we go to, the younger we tell them, the better.

I got married again in 2012. My husband is living with HIV and was diagnosed in the 80s, so he's lived with it for thirty years now. He's white British and I met him in London through a support group. We both work full-time and we're fine. My ambitions now would be to get a degree so I can get a better paid job, and just have a good life, see my son grow up and see him get married, settle down, have children. I'd like to see that my relationship with my husband is stable, and carries on the way it is carrying on now. I'm just hoping for a long life, I'm looking forward to retirement and getting old and volunteering and keeping myself busy. So, I don't think like, 'Oh, I only have a few years', I think I'm normal, like a normal person would be thinking. I am very grateful to the team at the Royal Free Hospital for supporting me through a very tough time during my diagnosis.

After the doctor told me about support groups, I started going to several of them and I found it's very important, I'd recommend it for anyone diagnosed with HIV. Either have a peer mentor, someone who will sit with you and talk to you, or go to support groups where you can talk about issues. When you see other people, it makes you more confident. You think, 'I'm not the only one', the support is fantastic, it really helped me, and it helped my son as well.

I just felt that there was a sheet of glass between me and the rest of the world.

NAME: RUTH
AGE: 70
DATE OF DIAGNOSIS: 8 MARCH 2002

I was born in 1947 in London. When I was about five my father, who worked for the Trade Commission, got a job in Lahore, Pakistan. My parents, my brother and I all went to live there, and after that we lived in Chittagong until I was 10, when I was sent to an all-girls direct grant grammar school in Bournemouth. I had quite a privileged education really, but I was at boarding school, which had all kinds of long-term effects on me.

I was always homesick to start with because we only saw our parents once a year. We were flown out to them, and by that time they were in Sri Lanka. But, the rest of the time we just spent at other schools or with our parents' friends. We didn't have much of a family life really. But after I got over my homesickness, I actually loved the school. Then my parents moved to Canada and they said, "We're missing you, why don't you leave boarding school, we're now in Canada and you could come to university here?" So I went to university in Canada, and, although there were many things I liked about it, I didn't feel at home. I did the first two years at Carlton University in Ottawa, then the second two years in the University of Saskatchewan, which was right in the middle of the prairies. I studied English and when I finished my degree in 1967 my friends in Canada were already dropping acid, listening to The Beatles and running away to San Francisco. But I decided that I could not settle permanently in Canada and I wanted to come home to England. So I came home to England on my own. My brother is still there.

Almost immediately I threw myself into the alternative scene in London. I was always looking for another home, another family. I became part of the libertarian left. I lived in squats, I became political. We wanted to try to live a different way and I started my sexual life in that milieu. We never practised safe sex in those days. We just tried to avoid becoming pregnant, but it was a totally alien environment for any notion of safer sex partly because there was as yet no HIV. It was also a real revolt against the nuclear family, and living in couples – so I never got married, I lived with boyfriends and had long-term partners. As a result of one of those I had a son in 1976, who is now grown up and a teacher and he lives nearby.

So that happened, and then my lifestyle changed, that whole collective way of life changed and I, like many others, started to live in a more individualistic way. I went to the London School of Economics, studying Social Policy as a postgraduate and I started to try to get a better life for me and my son, because I was now a single mum. Basically, I then started getting better jobs, and gradually I came to work in the voluntary sector. I worked in a psychotherapy centre for seven years, first as an information officer then I moved into finance and fundraising. After seven years I left that and I went to work at a regional health authority and then for a sexual health charity.

After I split up from my son's father I had a couple of short-term relationships but then, for many years, I had none at all. Partly this was because my son became quite troubled when I brought a boyfriend into our life together. Partly it was because supporting my son and making a living took up most of my time. I quickly stopped having relationships with anyone. I just focused on my work and making a nice life for him and I was celibate for about fourteen years. It was when he was in his late teens, and I was working in this sexual health charity, that I met the person who infected me.

I thought, 'I've had no relationships, nothing, for so long, now is my time'. I met a man through mutual friends. I found him attractive and we got involved. We were together for about two and a half years, and then we split up, which I took badly because I hadn't been in a relationship for so long. Then, a little while later I heard that he was ill with pneumonia and been admitted to hospital. I visited him and was shocked by his appearance. He looked extremely ill. I couldn't believe that pneumonia could do that to someone. I Googled it and found out that a particular type of pneumonia could be an indicator of AIDS. I began to be afraid, and eventually phoned the local sexual health clinic who advised me to go in for a test.

I asked a friend to come with me, who said, "Don't be silly – you're being paranoid. People like you don't get HIV." But she did come with me, and I was told a week later, on 8 March 2002, International Women's Day, that I had tested positive. I was in complete shock when I was diagnosed, like everyone is. I just felt that there was a sheet of glass between me and the rest of the world, between me and 'normal' people, and I could never go back through it. I used to look through it and see everybody leading their lives, and wish I could be on the other side of that glass. I began to see a therapist and I remember once driving up to the therapist's and behind me as I was parking were this whole family getting out of a campervan, and they were all laughing and chattering, and they looked so much like they were on the other side of plate glass, and I could never be where they were ever again.

I was working for a sexual health charity, and my doctor said, "You should take some time to come to terms with this, it is a tremendous shock." He wrote me a certificate for a viral infection and said to take two weeks off. My line manager at the place where I worked wasn't satisfied with that. She said, "What exactly have you got?" She really objected to the fact that I wouldn't tell her. She tried to coax the truth out of me by saying things like "Well it can't be cancer, because you'd be having appointments at the hospital." She was clearly trying to work out what I had. After I returned to work following some time off to visit the clinic, she sat me down and said, "I want to talk to you. Are you a danger to yourself? Are you a danger to others?" It was like she was finding out whether I had TB or some other notifiable disease that had to be reported to the NHS.

A couple of weeks later, after I had declined to tell her what I had, she produced a proposal to restructure the organisation including the single change that deleted my post. So I was made redundant. When I contacted the Terrence Higgins Trust for advice, I was told to be cautious about telling her I had HIV, which was the standard advice at the time. I didn't tell her. Maybe if I had the outcome would have been different. I was not thinking clearly. My father had died just before my diagnosis, and now I was facing losing my job.

I did consult a lawyer, but he said my chances were 50/50, so I did not fight the redundancy. I simply tried to get a fair settlement. I didn't tell the lawyer I had HIV, for the same reason I didn't tell my employer, so he couldn't use that in my defence. I lost my job, and was unemployed for about six months, not knowing what the future held.

Generally, I was in good health. I don't remember having any seroconversion illness. If I had I would've just thought of it as flu. My viral load at diagnosis wasn't enormously high; I didn't go on medication for about eight years. Which of course wouldn't happen now. The thinking at the time was to delay medication as long as possible, to avoid any adverse side effects, whereas now it's different. After eight years I got shingles and I became very thin, and my CD count was really low so that's when I started medication.

About six months after I was made redundant I found another job, which saved me really. I think it was the best thing I could've done, the best thing for my mental health. It was a job I enjoyed. It was all about patient participation in the NHS. I got on well with the people I worked with and made good friends. This time I told my line managers that I had HIV because I trusted them and they were understanding and helpful. I thought, 'I'm going to have to take time off to go to clinics, so they're going to have to know'. I didn't tell any of my work colleagues though. I didn't see any need to tell them.

Later on, because I was working on patient participation, I was asked to set up and support an HIV User Forum, for the local Primary Care Trust. It was for people who were HIV positive, to enable them to have a voice in local decision-making. I thought it was important to tell them that I was HIV positive too because I thought it would change how they saw me, as someone like them and not as someone patronising them.

Telling my son and the rest of the family is another story. On the day I was diagnosed, I phoned a 'helpline' from one of the leaflets I'd been given. The man on the other end of the phone said I should tell my family straight away. I was very suggestible because I had just been diagnosed and this was somebody I trusted. So when my son came in to the kitchen that afternoon, straight from the gym, I told him. I hadn't processed it myself yet. He just gave me an enormous hug.

He's always been supportive. There have been moments when he's been worried. He immediately got himself tested just to make sure I hadn't given it to him, and his girlfriend did as well. I understand that, but once, when I had a cut, and was looking after the grandchildren he said, "Mum, can you please cover that up?" and that hurt me a bit. But I understand it as well.

I'm not yet open about my HIV, although all my good friends know. My brother knows, but I never told my mother (my father had died before I was diagnosed). I didn't see any reason to tell her. She died in 2005, at the age of eighty-six. I felt that would have been a terrible thing to do to her.

As I woman, I look at my diagnosis this way: I hadn't had sex for many years before I met the man who infected me. Since being diagnosed fifteen years ago, I haven't been in a sexual relationship. But I think about the prejudice and now I'm pretty much resigned to the fact that I'll never have a relationship again. If I did tell a heterosexual man, I fear I would get a negative response. Of course, there is prejudice against gay men who are HIV positive too but I remember something that someone said in a meeting very recently, which was that sometimes when one HIV positive gay man tells another that he's positive, the response could well be 'me too', whereas in the white heterosexual world, which I'm in, it's very unlikely that the other would say 'me too'.

The other thing is the 'post-feminist' assumption that a 'real feminist' is feisty, assertive, sticks up for herself, and would never let anybody have sex with her without a condom. It's like, 'What kind of feminist are you that you let this happen to you?' So, you can't even be protected by the distorted kind of feminism that's around at the moment which is all about being a strong woman. I get the feeling that some women will want to know how I got it because they want to reassure themselves that they would never do the same.

When I was diagnosed, one of the phone numbers I called was Positively Women, because I thought of myself as a feminist and they were wonderful. They saved my life. I was a volunteer for them for many years. I wrote for the newsletter, I went on their volunteer training programme, I went to their weekly groups and I was on the management committee as well at some later point, as a user representative. But then they became Positively UK, and I disagreed with the way they went about that decision, and I resigned from the management committee. During the time I was involved with them they helped me feel like a normal person again. I gained a great deal from the women who worked and volunteered there.

I hadn't been involved in anything until I received the email about looking for volunteers for Positive Voices. I thought, it's time I did something again, so I joined up. What I find really shocking, which is what I say in Positive Voices all the time, and what I want to spend a lot more time thinking about, is that I had a very high-profile job giving presentations to health and youth work professionals, about the importance of safer sex, the importance of giving out the right messages. And all the time I was doing that, I was starting a relationship with someone where I was using no protection myself, absolutely none. That discordance between what I was saying, what I knew, and what I was actually doing, is, I think, really important to learn from. I feel it's not just about giving out information. That's what I want to say at Positive Voices. It's about valuing yourself, not making assumptions about other people and talking about sex more frankly. Because you never really know other people until, well, for a long time.

For example, when I told my friends I was embarking on a relationship for the first time in fourteen years, we never talked about whether I was protecting myself. Even at the age of fifty-one I was too embarrassed to walk into a chemist shop and look the cashier in the eye as I was buying condoms. You know, I actually felt ashamed of it. I was a fifty-one-year-old woman at the time, and yet I was personally really shy, about all sorts of things. I think that's an important message to get across.

If I could turn the clock back, would I do so? Of course I would. I definitely wouldn't like to be infected. I wish I wasn't. I can't understand anyone who says otherwise. Life teaches you things and of course you can derive something valuable from this just like you can from anything that happens to you. It'd be silly to say you couldn't but that doesn't mean I would want it if I could choose again.

That said, it has enlarged my life. I've met people from whom I've learnt a lot, a lot of gay men, and people from different backgrounds from me and I'm grateful for that, people I'd have never met otherwise, and who've been open and supportive and welcomed me. So that has been a real plus actually. I feel honoured and privileged to have met those people. I feel grateful for the opportunity to learn something about myself I suppose. It taught me a lesson. It continues to teach me a lesson, all the time, I keep thinking about what can I draw from this? What can I pass on? What will people find useful? What can they hear from my experience?

My friends thought I was going to die. Obviously, I told them because I wanted support from them, but I ended up being the supporter.

NAME: STEVE WALES
AGE: 39
DATE OF DIAGNOSIS: 22 JUNE 2007

I was born in Wales in 1978. I'm from Merthyr Tydfil. It's a depressed area and I remember the miners' strike, plus the poverty and disadvantage that came to such communities. From the age of four, when I started school, I was bullied until the day I left. I was known as 'Steven-Poof' from a very, very young age. In the area that I lived in, all sorts of labels are used frequently. It's very sad.

Between the ages of seven and eleven I was sexually abused by a family member and that sort of defined me for a number of years; I've had some real issues with forming relationships, friendships and trusting people, particularly men. I knew from a young age that I was gay. I also knew that what was being done to me was wrong, but I didn't have the confidence or the skills to challenge it.

I didn't have a very good relationship with my father and it's not that good now. He also used to taunt me and call me, 'Daddy's little girl'. My relationship with him was not great, and then obviously I was troubled by my sexuality, and the constant bullying and taunting. When I was eighteen I went to university in Cardiff, where there was a massive gay community, and I thought that it would be the making of me. It wasn't really. I was used and abused by men. I thought that – because of what happened to me as a child – the only way I could get somebody to love me was to be submissive. That happened so many times. I almost became a slut, and I don't mind using that word. That's what I referred to myself as. I was basically told by so many people that, "If you do this or that maybe

229

your relationship will develop", but that never happened.

I was a child in the AIDS epidemic, so I don't really remember the early horror stories in the mid to late 80s and the media campaign with the tombstones and things. By the early 90s I was a bit older and I was reading newspapers. I remember images on the front page of the red-tops about Kenny Everett dying, Freddie Mercury dying, and Elton John being a massive advocate for the sector. When I started having sex I was terrified of acquiring HIV.

Men would tell me that 'yes' they tested regularly, and it was safe to have bareback (i.e. condomless) sex. I believed them because I wanted to be loved, I wanted to feel normal, I wanted a relationship with a man to be nice. I was silly, and I believed what they said.

I found out I was HIV positive following a routine blood donation. I used to donate blood every six months and I was quite big on that. I've got a rare blood group. Before I contracted HIV, my blood could be given to anybody, so I was really big on donating blood. So there was a six-month window for me to have acquired HIV, between donating blood the last time and the next donation where it was screened, and that's how I was diagnosed.

I was diagnosed at 4:15pm on 22 June 2007. I acquired the virus in Gran Canaria. I went on a bit of a 'weekend-offenders' holiday to an all-inclusive gay resort. It was because of my behaviour at that time: too much sun, too much sangria and too much sex. The diagnosis itself was horrendous, I received a letter from the Welsh blood donor service asking me to contact them, which I did. I spoke to a member of their staff and they told me that they'd entered me into a survey and would I like to be part of that survey? I agreed, and I had to make an appointment to see them. When I got there, there was no survey. I arrived with my letter, all excited to be part of some new blood service initiative. I was led into what seemed like a large boardroom and was left in there for around fifteen minutes, then in came a female. I don't know whether she was a doctor or a nurse – I couldn't tell you. She sat down, her body language was dreadful, and she gave me the diagnosis. By that time, it was 4:30 on 22 June 2007. I went away with a Post-It note on which was written the telephone number for the HIV clinic at the University of Wales, Cardiff, and was told to give them a ring on Monday. Then that was me, out the door. I got in my car and a poignant song came on, I thought it was like something from a bloody movie. R.E.M's 'Everybody Hurts'. It was blaring, and I totally broke down. How I got home I can't say. I drove straight to ASDA and I bought a litre of vodka and I just got pissed. That whole weekend is a total blur. I don't know how I got up on the Monday morning and went to work. I looked at that Post-It note every day for four months and never did anything with it.

Four months after diagnosis I told my two best friends in a drunken stupor. When I made my disclosure, I was hysterical, I was crying, I could hardly get my words out. They responded in the same way. Having a diagnosis of HIV when you live in the Welsh valleys, or when you lived in the Welsh valleys ten years ago, means that lots of people are uneducated about blood-borne viruses etc, they still think HIV is as bad now as it was in 1982. Knowing what I know now, I think if you tell somebody with confidence that you're living with HIV and they ask you questions and you're informed, they seem to deal with it a lot better.

My friends thought I was going to die. Obviously, I told them because I wanted support from them, but I ended up being the supporter. I honestly thought of never telling anyone again. Obviously, I had to but I had the same response from my mother. She said, "Don't tell anybody about this. Don't tell your sister, don't tell your father, nobody needs to know, this is going to bring shame on the family."

So again, I was devastated, I just told the three closest people to me that I was HIV positive and I've had this horrendous reaction. I felt dirty, I almost felt that you only had to look at me and I could infect you, it was awful. Eventually I rang the number and spoke to a HIV specialist at the hospital in Cardiff and made an appointment to go and see him the next day. That was the longest twenty-four hours of my life. Obviously, I knew I was HIV positive, I'd had the diagnosis. I'd had at least three horrendous experiences with disclosure, I was terrified of what was going to happen to me in the hospital.

The HIV clinic is in the worst place possible. I just kept thinking that somebody was going to see me sat there in the infectious clinic. Your name would be called over the tannoy. I only went to two or three appointments and I was prescribed Atripla. It gave me the most morbid dreams, I couldn't think rationally, I had some bad gastro and incontinence issues. I articulated this to the doctors and they were like, "This is the wonder drug, this is the single pill, you are lucky that we are prescribing it. If you don't take this, you are going to die." So I took the conscious decision to die. I couldn't cope mentally, I couldn't cope physically. I couldn't cope with the medication, couldn't cope with the stigma of being HIV, terrified of the stigma of being exposed in my community.

I needed somebody basically to tell me that everything was going to be OK. I needed a hand. I work in the sector myself now, it's the first thing I do because that's what they want. I know you're supposed to have professional boundaries, but I really don't begrudge anybody a cuddle if that's what they want, you know, because that's what some people need.

I never went back to the clinic until November 2015, when I was very, very, very unwell. I had a CD4 count of twenty-nine. I'd lived without medication for seven years and I was ready to die. Although I knew that death was going to catch up to me, I'd just buried HIV. I almost filed it away. Anything on the TV about AIDS, HIV, sexual health, I would simply turn the TV over. It was awful, reflecting back now, because I pretty much lost eight years of my life. I let HIV define me and control me, where I should've taken the bull by the horns and turned it on its head and embraced it, really.

I told one other person – my closest friend. I met her in my church. I come from quite a religious family, and although I drifted away I did like attending our church, which is a beautiful building. I would sit at the back and she would be at the back as well and we would look at each other and smile. That happened for about three months, so we started sitting in closer pews until eventually we were sitting next to each other. The most beautiful friendship formed. I'm thirty-nine now, Michelle's forty-three, so there's four years between us. She's a Macmillan nurse.

I eventually told her, and she was absolutely brilliant. She found me the most discreet clinic in the Royal Glamorgan Hospital in Llantrisant. She made an appointment for me to go there, no waiting time, I went straight in with the nurse-specialist and the consultant. This was in November 2015. I met the most amazing nurse, she was a proper 'Valleys woman', calling me 'Love' and giving me the cuddles that I wanted. I didn't ask for them, she knew that I needed them. From the moment that I went there it changed my life.

Between November and January there was a two-month period when I started taking ART. I began to realise how poor my mental health was. The ART started to build me up, physically and mentally. I was on antibiotics though, because my CD4 took a long time to start to improve. It's still plateaued now at around about 270. It's never got any better. I started talking about my condition a lot more and had counselling sessions with Michelle who I met at the church. She built my confidence and my self-esteem, it was just amazing. Then I found the Terrence Higgins Trust online peer-support community.

My line of work for a number of years was community regeneration. I worked for the voluntary council for Gwent and worked alongside the local authority, and the county borough council to regenerate disadvantaged communities utilising European funding. But I became aware that I wanted to support people with HIV and in March 2016, I was employed full-time by the Terrence Higgins Trust. I was doing online peer-support and I've never looked back. I'd always known what the Trust was, but I was afraid of those three letters: H-I-V. I knew that if I engaged with THT then I had to address my HIV.

I also found out about the Long Term Survivors' Group. I went for a weekend retreat with them in March 2016 and I came away from there feeling so empowered, so inspired. I was talking to people who had lived with HIV in the 80s and had taken the horrible AZT, and the horrific side effects that they'd had through the medication. The appalling stigma and discrimination they faced, not just from society as a whole but also from medical professionals.

I left Terrence Higgins Trust in February this year, because I did at that point feel a little bit 'HIV-d out'. I'd been working full time in the sector and doing lots of volunteering. I thought to myself that I wanted to remain with the Trust but not in a paid capacity. I could do more in my peer-support role, rather than as just one of their staff. My current employment is in substance abuse and sexual health, supporting people with Hepatitis-C. But I can now confidently say to my clients, if it's appropriate to do so, "You're not on your own, I'm HIV positive, I can support you."

When I talk to people with HIV I tell them to live their dreams. To not be afraid of the virus. To engage with services. Not to make the mistakes that I made. I was sat in the room when a seventeen-year-old boy was diagnosed. It was the most horrific experience of my life. How I composed myself I don't know. His parents were there, they didn't care about the HIV, they were ashamed that he was gay. He had been abused and I believe in my heart that he was infected on purpose. But he also inspired me, because he kept his prescription, he started taking his medication, and he's getting on with life. I think maybe he was a lot more confident because he was younger. I did a lot of motivational work with him, giving emotional support, providing information. He was brilliant. People like that make me want to continue doing what I do.

I would say the stigma of living with a blood-borne illness is the biggest issue now for people living with HIV. The damage I did to my body will never be reversible. It has left me with some memory loss – my short-term memory is horrific. But my long-term memory is brilliant. I did the dementia test and everything. I actually scored twenty-eight out of thirty, so I'm not that bad. Sometimes I talk to people and for the life of me I can't think of their name. So, HIV has left me with some physical damage that's non-reversible. But, obviously, I'm medicated and undetectable. The medication is obviously effective. I do have some side effects, but when I'm working with people I tell them that side effects are not compulsory, you are in charge. If you're not getting along with your medication you tell your consultant and you tell them you want something different.

Whatever I can do to raise awareness about anything to do with sexual health, particularly HIV, then I do. I think that's a big part of challenging the stigma. We need to get lay-members of society to know that HIV is not something to be scared of. "I can't pass it on, I'm not infectious." I always tell my clients, that message. "Keep taking your medication, remain undetectable. You can have the same, if not a healthier, life, than somebody who is negative."

Because of the attention I get, I go to my clinic every three months, they test me for everything. Glucose, cholesterol; if something is wrong with my physical health it would probably be picked up before somebody who's negative. They don't have the same level of care.

What I'm most mindful of is that you need to have a healthy mental state of affairs. I'm a trained mindfulness facilitator. I did a course earlier this year to deliver mindfulness sessions, and it works. I'm not saying that you should only have complementary therapy, but I think if you've got a healthy mind towards your HIV diagnosis then you can be visible in your community and you're normalising your condition. Until more people who are living with HIV do that, then the stigma is going to remain.

My dream job would be working for a humanitarian organisation working in sub-Saharan Africa dealing with HIV. Not just working directly with people who are living with it and affected by it, but challenging drug companies, challenging governments and those companies to end stigma.

What would stop me? Nothing would stop me. I'm constantly looking, and if something comes up like that then I would up-sticks and go. I'm also thinking, probably not this year or next year but the year after, hopefully I'll be able to apply for a sabbatical. If I couldn't find a paid role then I would be happy to do it in a voluntary capacity for a few months; whatever is needed.

At the moment I don't have a partner. When I thought that I was toxic I was terrified of having sex, absolutely terrified. But, now I look at life differently. I have been dating. It's been on my terms. I've been in control, I don't allow men to manipulate me anymore. I'm honest from the outset: "I'm HIV positive, if you have an issue with that's your issue. I'm happy to sit and talk those issues through with you. But, if you're that prejudiced that you don't want the conversation then I don't want you as part of my life."

I think there are things in life that make us or break us and it's different for every individual. This was my kind of Damascene moment, or whatever we want to call it.

NAME: ESTHER DIXON-WILLIAMS
AGE: 42
DATE OF DIAGNOSIS: 1 NOVEMBER 2013

I'm 42. I was diagnosed with HIV on November 11, 2013. I contracted HIV during August 2013 either on the 13th or 14th. I was seeing one person, so it was very clear to me when it happened.

I had the weirdest flu. It was summertime, and I didn't understand what was going on. I got a rash, and I didn't understand why I had flu. I'd never had experienced an STI so I didn't think to link it to being exposed to HIV, even thought these were all classic signs of HIV transmission. When I felt ill after that weekend, my friend said to me – and this was before the two weeks before I had the flu – 'you should go and get PEP within seventy-two hours if you feel you've been exposed', and I was like, 'No, I don't think I've been exposed'. But then it just kind of niggled at me. I've gone for a sexual health check-up since I was 21, probably about once every two or three years. I've always said, 'Test me for everything'. I have always preferred to know if there was anything that would need to be managed.

So I went to the clinic and a week later they called me, and they said, 'Can you come in tomorrow?' and I said, 'I can't really'. Because I lived about twenty minutes away I said 'I'll jump in the car and come down now. What do you need to tell me?' They said, 'You need to speak to a doctor, and you need to come in tomorrow'. All the hairs on the back of my neck went up. I got really serious with the woman on the phone, and I said 'Look, you cannot call me at 4:30 in the afternoon, tell me to come in the next day, because I have to see a doctor and not explain what's going on. I'm going to give you the opportunity now to put down the phone, go and speak to somebody, and call me back with the information that you need to give me'. And she was like 'Oh we don't do this stuff on the phone' and I wasn't going to take no for an answer, I stated 'You need to tell me what's going on'. My mind was racing and I thought she was going to tell me it was syphilis, gonorrhea or something like that. I didn't have any symptoms, but it never for a minute crossed my mind that it could be HIV.

So she called me back and she said, 'Look, I'm really really sorry, you have HIV'. So, I thought, 'What the hell is going on here?' I was shocked. But because I've worked in a sector were there are crises all the time I tend to be incredibly calm in emergency situations.

What I needed were facts. I had a couple of gay friends with HIV, I had friends with HIV/AIDS in the 90s, so I understood a bit, but I didn't really know that much. I went to this clinic – and it was awful. I had a nurse who spoke at a hundred miles an hour, so I was saying, 'Now look, if you want to give me information, you need to slow down so that I can understand the information that you are giving me. If you're not able to do that then remove yourself from the room, and go and get another member of staff to come and speak with me'. I just got, really serious.

I wanted the clear information and all the doctors I met in those first three months were terrified of me! A friend came with me to the first few appointments said, 'You need to relax', because she said 'I looked like was ready to jump over the desk and strangle them!'

Then I met with the consultant, who said to me, 'You're in primary infection', which I knew. I gave him the date I contracted the virus and he was really shocked that I knew the date. He said, 'There's something else going on, because you don't have a viral load, and you're supposed to have the highest viral load now'. My viral load was undetectable, and it's been like that ever since. I've had a blip where it went up to three hundred copies and then four hundred copies and then it dropped back to zero again. So if the trend continues then I will be deemed a long-term non-progressive, which there is little research on and has it own set of issues. It was a complete roller coaster. You have HIV but you're naturally controlling it. I'd never heard of this before.

I started speaking to the Terrence Higgins Trust because I thought, 'OK, I need to meet other people'. I knew through the work that I did that in these kinds of situation you need to find the rest of your tribe. Then you need to pick out the members of the tribe that you get on naturally with. Then you need to increase your learning and understanding. So that's what I did. .

I watched all the HIV/AIDS documentaries. *We Were Here*, *How to Survive a Plague*, *The Normal Heart*. I watched documentaries, films and read everything and anything. I quickly found out there was a lot of nonsense and misinformation online and it was probably the worst place to try and find information with no knowledge.

I thought I need to learn more, so then I found AIDS Map/ NAM, I found I-Base, I found UK-CAB – which was a community activist and advocacy group. I got a counsellor, and we had a phone session once a week for the first nine months and then after that it was once every two weeks until we finished. Counselling was the biggest help.

I was in physiological survival mode at that time and maybe that's because I had worked with people who were stuck – really stuck. I know through the work I do that people will meet one challenging life event and will become stuck with it as a result. It can be a horrific life event, a very difficult life event but I knew that whatever happened, I couldn't get stuck.

The first six months to probably eight months I was unpacking how I felt about it, how to get stronger, how to be comfortable about it, how to understand my new normal and how to function – I mean I took a new job, I started a new post two weeks after diagnosis. I was just like 'Let's just keep this moving'. I established that a) it's not the 80s: there are ARVs and b) I'm not going to die. So I decided that I'm not going to take time off work, because it's just not going to help.

I realised I had to get myself together. I had to work, figure this out and move on. Because if I didn't figure this out, it could just floor me and I wasn't sure when I would get up again. I'm not critical of those people who it has floored, we all deal with things in different ways, but I was determined. That said, I was depressed at times; not deep depression but I would get kind of a cloud every so often, and be really sad about it. I kind of wanted kids, but never had done anything enough to have kids. The diagnosis came in a time in my life where I was contemplating 'where am I going? I'm about to be forty. Is this the career I want to be in? Do I want to change? Do I really want kids?' If I really wanted kids then I needed to meet someone, and then this came and completely took me off my feet and changed the whole dynamic.

I started to meet other people living with HIV. They were living amazing lives, they were living normally – whatever normal is. It didn't impact them anymore. That said, I didn't disclose to many people and felt I would take my time to do so. I'm just approaching that place now, four years later, where if someone was to find out I don't really care, this is who I am. I went to train for the UK community advisory board. I met some really good people, many who are still friends of mine, on that training course. I met some women and they had been living with HIV for 20 to 25 years and they were just really inspiring. It made me realise, 'You know what, I've got this – it's going to be OK'. I started to learn about activism,

HIV activism, how this whole thing goes on, and the history, but I was still incredibly green. But I came back feeling really liberated and feeling, 'OK, there's much more to all this and there's actually this whole world that I've never known'. The world of advocacy and dealing with pharmaceutical companies, clinicians, governments and the regulators. I also learnt that I would become an advocate.

I realise that actually I'm much more interested in the scientific side of HIV and areas such as drug development, pharmacokinetics, the short term and the long-term side effects of drugs and impact on long term conditions as we age. I'm also interested in the fact that there's little data for women and the long-term effects for taking antiretrovirals for life and the different stages in a woman life so, there are still a lot of unanswered questions. The concerns I have now with regard to advocacy is the rising and unmanaged epidemic in East Europe and Central Asia, continuing lack of access in many parts of Africa and growing drug resistant to first line antiretrovirals. This is also coupled with the fact that there has never been universal access of ARV's worldwide.

My health now is fine. It took me a while to understand completely that seeing my HIV consultant once a year is reasonable, but that's all they want to see you, once a year. But when I look back, nearly four years later, I'm very grateful for the experience, and I'll stay grateful. I wouldn't change it – it's made me who I am and is part of my identity. This virus is here to stay and it's cool, we will co-exist.

I think there are things in life that make us or break us and it's different for every individual. This was my kind of Damascene moment, or whatever we want to call it. It has been difficult, but I've come out swinging. I mean, it's not often that I reflect on everything that's happened. But it's been an incredible four years.

In a weird and twisted way, pardon the pun, I get out of bed a lot more positive these days.

NAME: JAMES ISAACS
AGE: 28
DATE OF DIAGNOSIS: 15 JULY 2014

I grew up in the country, just outside London, in Hemel Hempstead. I moved to London about eight years ago after going through schooling, and a brief stint touring the world as a musician. I was in two bands, and at one point one of those bands took me to far-flung places such as India, doing stadium tours on the tops of mountains, down by the Himalayas. At that time, I was still at school, I was in my final year. The band took over, and in 2007 we played 158 shows.

I'm now twenty-eight. My music career came to an end in about 2010, and then a year later I moved to London. What prompted the move was that I wanted my own independence. I'd not long come out as gay. I felt that I needed some space to learn about myself. My family split when I was four and both my parents remarried, so I had to do the whole coming-out thing twice. With one set of parents, then moving in with the other set of parents at a later date, and having to do the whole thing again. My move in with my other parents was not spurred on by a bad acceptance or reaction to me coming out; it was just what it was at the time.

I was diagnosed with HIV on 15 July 2014. I'd been in quite an abusive relationship, emotionally and mentally, sometimes physically, for about a year, with somebody I was head over heels in love with. Eventually I had a mental breakdown and I got away from him. I went to a standard sexual health screening three months later, as I was sort of getting myself on my feet again. I was in south London at about two o'clock on a Monday afternoon, when I received the call. They said, "Oh, we need you to come in." I got off the phone, on what was a hot summer's day, feeling very cold.

It wasn't a shock but only for one reason, and that was because four days previously I'd just returned to work after three months off. And on the same day I received a call from my abusive ex, who said, "Well, I finally went and got tested", and I kind of went, "Hang on, what do you mean 'finally'?" Because for the year we were together, every time I went and got tested, which was every three months, he would go and get tested at his clinic at the same time. Or so I thought. It turns out he never did, he would fake it and have a pint somewhere.

So he said, "I finally went and got tested, and my results have come back positive for several things." I was, at this point, awaiting my test results, so I was expecting it.

We hadn't had sex for about six months, but towards the end of our relationship, and in the course of one very heated argument, it just happened. It was more bordering on rape. Weeks later I was then very, very ill in bed with what I thought was the flu. It was a week before coming off work for a week's holiday, and during that time – which I later found was my seroconversion – I was forced by my employer to work through it.

Anyway, four days later I found out I was HIV positive. The first day back at work, four members of my team were signed off due to stress. I had thirty-seven staff working underneath me, a few million pounds to bring in and I'd just found this out. I still wasn't quite with it, it was a very significant knock to my mental stability. I was feeling very nervous, anxious and agitated constantly, and with all that on my back I thought, 'I need to tell someone at work'.

So I disclosed within twenty-four hours of finding out to my area manager and it was handled, on the face of it, very well I thought. Except three weeks later, I was called in to a room and essentially pushed into accepting a cut to my responsibilities and a dock to my pay because my hours were being cut down to eight hours per week. I loved my job, so for me it was a big knock.

Their reason for doing it was, 'We don't think you're coping, we want to give you some time to come to terms with it, before we put your hours back up'. Which obviously at the time I felt, 'OK, I don't want any more time off, but I feel like I've got to accept I'm going to lose everything I worked for'.

After that, the next week I was very, very low. I was feeling like I was losing it in terms of control. To me that was the turning point. I went to the Bloomsbury Clinic in London, and they've got patient representatives who are employed by the clinic and are living and have been living with HIV for a number of years. They know what it feels like. I went in and had a chat with them one day and a week later, I bounced back. To me, it was very much a case of, 'I'm ready for this, I'm ready to take control again'.

Something needed to change, so I quit my job. Having found just how much I valued my mental health, having lost it for a portion of the year before, I couldn't do that again. By that point I had already started my medication and that was going OK. For the next year I was living with friends, trying to find a job. I came out through social media, as HIV positive, on 2 October 2014. I felt that by being open and honest, instead of living in fear of my HIV, I could actually use this to own it and educate others.

I decided I wanted to be public with it quite early on anyway, earlier on than that, but I held back. In terms of expectations, it was more raising awareness that, after my diagnosis, I learned quite quickly that my level of education regarding HIV versus what I knew before, and versus what most people my age at that time knew, was completely warped. Now it was a case of, 'God, if only I'd known that before' or, 'Oh my God, this is insane. Why do we not teach this? Why do we not educate this? If we did this, we could really challenge the stigma'.

I'd been trying to find the right words to use to come out with for a while and what did it in the end was meeting up with my old trumpet player from my band, after about three years, for a drink. This was the beginning of October, having been diagnosed in July, so it was three months apart. Within ten minutes of turning up, he'd cracked a joke about the fact that I'd now come out as gay, and another one – a very bad joke – about catching HIV or AIDS, developing AIDS. So I just turned it around on him and said, "Just so you know, I was diagnosed three months ago with HIV", and for the next three hours he couldn't figure out if I was playing the most warped joke on him, or whether I was actually being serious.

We ended up having a very good evening actually, but on my journey home I dropped him a text, which read along the lines of, 'I've had a pretty bad year, but if you can't look back at it and say you've lived and learnt from it, then what point is there in saying that you've both lived life, and enjoyed it? I'm HIV positive yes, but I'm still me and I have every intention of outliving all of you, as gracefully and disgracefully as possible, learn to live, laugh, love and carry on'. I realised after that, all of a sudden, that those were the words I'd been looking for. So I just copied that, popped it onto social media, and went to bed.

The afternoon of the next day I got a phone call from my mother. She just said, "What have you done?" Earlier on in my diagnosis I'd said to her, "Look, I want to be quite public with this" because I wanted to use it as an educational tool. I don't think she realised just how public I meant. All of a sudden, my cousins and my aunts and my uncles who'd seen this got in touch with her and said, "What's going on?"

The positive outcomes that came from this were twofold. Some of them were people I'd known in my past, people who I'd gone to school with, who'd read that and gone, "Oh, wow", but also, "Oh wow, I didn't realise that, you sound like you've accepted it, I'm reading this from someone I know and they don't sound scared, that's different." So I opened up a dialogue.

The other thing was the number of people who got in touch; people I didn't know and people I did, and had in some cases known for many years, who had never told anyone about their own diagnosis. That surprised me quite a lot.

Do I notice stigma? I think that there's definitely a lot of stigma still around. I haven't seen it face to face and haven't had much experience with it personally myself. I think that's another reason why I decided to come out quite so publicly, because a lot of stigma is formed by a fear of the unknown. Stigma is a big fear of something scary that you don't quite know all the facts about. A lot of that is based around fear from other people, third party fear.

There was a very real sense of fear in the 1980s, with the falling tombstones advert and all that. It was in the public consciousness because it was such a striking campaign. A lot of people look back on that, especially HIV positive people, and say, "God, that's done so much damage" but actually, if you're looking at it at the time, the message was, 'This is something really scary and real, we don't know why people are dropping down dead, you need to know about it', and the best way to do that is to strike fear in to people. It was a successful campaign for what it was.

I think a lot of people paint it in a different colour than it should be. It's a debate about their own bias and identity. And if you look at HIV in the last thirty years, and where we've come in that time, there's no other field of medicine that's moved that fast. Also the level of education that's gone along with it; when you look at schools where sexual health education wasn't compulsory – well, it is now.

I'm a part of Positive Voices and we talk about how normal a life with HIV can be and also how important it is to get testing in, to normalise testing and to actually not fear it. In a weird and twisted way, pardon the pun, I get out of bed really a lot more positive these days. Only because I think a diagnosis, whether it's HIV or something else, a very life- changing diagnosis, makes you wake up and you realise and value what you have in your life, what you want in your life and what you do with your life. So that, from a mental health perspective actually, is a twist to how most people perceive the diagnosis of, 'Oh my god'.

It took a little while to get there, but that's where I am today. I think what my diagnosis taught me more than anything, that I've noticed before and after, is instead of getting up and living my life and emulating what I wanted and who I wanted to be, I now get up and I am who I want to be and do what I want to do.

My current employer has been fantastic. On my first day working as a deputy manager for a retail unit in St Pancras, my new manager quit. I discovered six years' worth of paperwork not done, no organisation and I ended up hitting the ground running and fell into loving it. What was interesting was that on this occasion I decided to keep my mouth shut about my HIV status. I decided that I wanted to get past probation before saying it. A few months in to the job, I was taken in to see the HR manager and my area manager. I thought, 'Oh, I'm getting my promotion already!' Then they said, "We hear that you've got a slight illness." I thought, 'The one time I kept my mouth shut'.I haven't been keeping my mouth shut but this time I did and they found out via Google.

I thought, 'OK, let's turn this around', so I said, "Let's have an open discussion, don't feel afraid to ask me any questions, I won't judge you. Yes, I'm HIV positive, ask away." I think what helped was that they had never ever had this situation where someone had come out as positive, or they'd been faced with this. They'd seen how hard-working I was and from what they had seen of me they had no idea that I had a chronic illness. I got the question, "But you don't look ill?" I didn't look ill. They'd seen that and they'd seen how hard I had worked before being met with, "Oh! You've got…oh, OK!" We had a good chat, and one of the questions that came up was, "Surely you should have told us? If you cut yourself while doing a delivery, surely you're a hazard to someone?" I let that one go, and very calmly said, "Well actually you know, my medication stops me from passing it on. If someone else cuts themselves I'd immediately want to clear that up with gloves on, because I could catch something from their blood."

By the end of that meeting one of them laughed and said, "We've really got the right guy", but a week later the question was raised about whether my colleagues should know. I stayed kind of quiet because I wanted to tell my team eventually. Again, it's a point of education. A week later my area manager came to visit me, and he said, "You know that meeting we had? Forget it ever happened." At that point they'd gone away, done a lot of research and realised how some of the questions they were asking were very out of line. At that point, they'd seen how well I had handled it in hindsight and realised, "OK, wow." Now my team all know, I haven't had one negative reaction; I've had some very positive reactions. I'm an open book for questions.

The prime message is twofold; one – don't be afraid to ask questions, don't live in fear of asking a question. Never put yourself in fear of gaining knowledge, or learning about something you don't know. But secondly – especially when we're talking about sexual health –looking after your sexual health isn't just about looking after you. It's about looking after your partner or partners. Sexual health doesn't need to be so scary. Just because you may not have talked about it in your life up until this point doesn't mean it should be a topic we don't talk about. It's just more normalising that so getting tested becomes more of a routine. At whatever point you are in life, whether you are younger or older, whether you're being promiscuous in your sex life or whether you're not, it's about looking after your health.

I'm now in a very happy, loving relationship but in the past if I met someone and I liked them I'd disclose to them straight away. I did that because if I was a HIV negative man, who had a fear of HIV and I found out I slept with somebody and they hadn't been open and honest, how would I feel then? I would probably feel angry; I would probably be in more fear than I was beforehand. Finding out afterwards is like finding out through a third party, whereas what I've done in previous relationships, whether casual or long term, is chosen to be honest and open from the start. At that point in time, if it's somebody whose knowledge is limited, you have a small window where you can actually educate them and they will listen. That window could be all it takes to help them learn, to help them change how they view their sexual health in the future.

To conclude, I think since diagnosis I've come to learn and accept myself. Past that, I think what I'm proud of since my diagnosis is how I'm finding it having a positive impact on helping other people realise that HIV positive people actually can live a normal live. You can be stigmatised by people who don't have it, and from people who do have it, like yourself. Self-stigma, in other words. Self-stigma is probably one of the bigger issues that isn't talked about at all.

People fear telling a parent, only to eventually tell them and have them say, "OK – we're still here." It's the same fear as coming out as gay or trans or even saying, "Mum, I've got pink hair!" Whatever it may be, it's a fear of coming out as something. It's a fear of rejection over something you can't change, something that is you.

All of a sudden, I felt in so much pain. If you've ever been in love and you've had your heart broken, it's that kind of suffering. You instantly want to be swallowed up whole by the universe, and to kind of disappear.

NAME: CHRIS ALDERTON
AGE: 28
DATE OF DIAGNOSIS: 14 JUNE 2015

I grew up in Suffolk. I have an older sister, an older brother and a younger brother who's got special needs. Mum and dad married very young and they're still together and happy, and still living in the house we grew up in.

At thirteen, I told my parents that I thought I was gay. They were really supportive. They said, "Let's see what happens" because I was quite young. Then when I was fifteen I came back to them and said "Yeah, I'm definitely gay", and that was it. It was easy.

I then left school at sixteen to go to college and studied child-care for two years. I wanted to work in nurseries, to be a pre-school practitioner – which is what they're called now. As I was studying I discovered I quite enjoyed working with new-borns and young children, so when I finished my studying at eighteen I went to work for a holiday company for four years, travelling all over Europe as a nanny.

I came back to the UK in 2011 and decided to get a job as a private nanny in London. Subsequently, I worked for a family who had twin girls. They had another baby soon after I started, so I was in charge of three under three. I loved it and stayed with them for about three years. I'm still in really good contact with them and I'm godfather to the children.

I did some more training and became a sleep trainer and a postnatal depression councillor. I rebranded myself into a twins and baby specialist and went to work for another family who had twins, nannying there for a year and a half while consulting on the side, teaching parents how to deal with their children's behaviour and what to do, feeding issues, anything like that. I started volunteering at Great Ormond Street Hospital, supporting patients and parents going through a difficult time and giving company to children who were living there and taking care of them so the parents could have some respite.

As a young gay guy living in London I had lots of different relationships. I was just exploring my sexuality. I've always been very open about sex and being sexual. I don't see it as a taboo thing, like many people. I went through most of my twenties really enjoying sex, being out there with lots of different partners and doing lots of different things. I think my longest relationship was probably a year, until I met my current partner, James, which has been four years now.

For years I kept getting recurring tonsillitis. I would be having weeks off work, being on antibiotics, and in one year, I had tonsillitis eight times. Eventually the NHS agreed to just remove them because they were just causing so much trouble. About six weeks after I had them out, I got ill again. I thought this is really weird – I'd just got back from a festival as well and thought maybe I'd just overdone it. Something was wrong, so I went back to the doctor's and they said, "We think you should have an HIV test, but we can't do it here because we don't have the capacity to do it, you need to go to a GUM clinic." I was like, "Fine, OK." I didn't know much about HIV, but I'd always been very good when it came to having STI tests after partners, every three months, every two months – I would go all the time.

So I went for some tests, and in my head I was convinced that it was not going to be HIV. I thought I might have chlamydia and it had been lying dormant. About a week later I got a call saying

I needed to come in and talk about my results. Even on the journey to the hospital I was like, "It won't be that."

It was 14 June 2015. I went into the room, and I hadn't even sat down and the guy said, "Your results have come back positive. You've got HIV." It was quite blunt and actually quite harsh. I don't know if whoever would have told me I would have reacted badly to. I guess there's no good way of ever giving that news to someone.

I just remember darkness overcoming my brain, it just being black and I couldn't see any light. I wanted the world to swallow me up. I had a million and one questions, I was panicking, I was hyperventilating, I actually got quite angry and tried to throw stuff at the guy. I was just so erratic. All of a sudden, I felt in so much pain. If you've ever been in love and you've had your heart broken, it's that kind of suffering. You instantly want to be swallowed up whole by the universe, and to kind of disappear.

I came out of there and had to go and have some bloods and stuff, and in that process I called my best friend, Steph. I was hysterically crying down the phone and I said, "This has happened, I need someone to come and meet me, I can't even function to get home." She got up and left work and came and met me and consoled me.

My first thought was that James had been unfaithful to me. I said, "He's lied to me, he's broken our trust." I thought he had done something to me. Then I thought, 'Well, how am I going to tell him anyway? How do you tell someone this?'

I called him, and said that he needed to come home from work early that day. Strangely enough on the journey I took home I actually bumped into him on one of the changeovers on the Underground.

He was like, "What's wrong, what's wrong?" and I said "Just wait till we get home." He was holding me and saying, "Just tell me, just tell me. Have you got cancer?" I said, "It would be easier if I told you I had cancer." So I just told him. He put his arms around me, hugged me, and said "Let's just get you home." We got home, we discussed our relationship and decided that neither of us had been unfaithful. I trusted him and he trusted me. The next step was, 'Oh god, what if he's got it?' He was tested and put on PEP, although they said, "Even if he did have it, this isn't going to work, because you've been having sex for years without a condom." He was told that in three months he would get a conclusive result to see if he was negative.

At that point our relationship was kind of in peril. I needed to work out what I was going to do and we were still in limbo with him. He needed my support, I needed his support, so we were just clashing. I really wasn't sure our relationship was going to survive at that point. Then his result came back and he was negative. This actually came as a bit of a power crush to me, because I was like, 'Crap, now I have to deal with it'. My job was a really good distraction for me, being a nanny. With children, you can't go into work sad and unhappy because they need your love and support. So when I was at work, I was totally fine. I wasn't even thinking about it.

After this point James was always calm, he never shouted and he never told me what I needed to do. He never told me how I needed to feel or anything, he just listened and supported. It must've been really hard on him because we hadn't told many people. That's the point that we decided to let him tell one of his close friends.

I'd told mum over the phone because I live in London and she's in Suffolk. She just said, "OK, we'll deal with this, we'll just get on with it." She's very much a stiff-upper-lip type. As long as it's not fatal, we can deal with it. She said something to me that I didn't understand, which I wasn't happy about then, but I get now. She said, "This has happened to someone like you because you're strong, and you're going to turn this into something amazing, I promise you." At that time, when you're three months into a diagnosis, it's not what you want to hear. But I really do get it now.

Work was OK but I felt myself going into a downward spiral outside of it. I started drinking quite a lot, taking drugs, just wanting to escape. I'd go out, and put myself in difficult situations. I was in self-destruct mode. Then, about three-and-a-half months in, I'd drunk quite a lot one night and came home really late one Friday morning. It must've been about 6.30am. James was leaving for work. He said, "You're a mess, you need to sleep, we'll deal with this when we get home."

I felt HIV was defining me. I couldn't remember my life before HIV, I couldn't remember any happy memories about my life, I couldn't remember meeting James, just complete darkness. I was hysterically crying, overcome with pain, just by myself at home, feeling like I was burdening everyone with my diagnosis. That I was dirty, that nobody would care about me. And I attempted to take my life. I just remember calling James, holding a knife and just being like – I don't know what I'm doing, I just don't want to be here. He was trying to get back and just calming me down but he couldn't get through to me. He hung up and I just had the knife in my hand, on my wrist. I was in so much pain; pain that I can't describe, it just seemed easier to go. Then my phone rang. It was my friend Steph. She was just chatting to me, really regularly, kind of just about her problems and work and stuff. She was distracting me; she told me to just go and lie down and close my eyes and she was going to talk to me, and I fell asleep. When I woke up James was there. He'd arrived home, and in the meantime he'd called Steph because he knew she could get through to me.

I'd hit rock bottom, and I knew that I could either choose to go, or start rebuilding my life. At this point I was actually changing jobs and I'd just got another job, three-and-a-half days nannying for a lovely family who I'm still currently with. But I was asking myself

–what's next? How do I start rebuilding my life? How to we rebuild our relationship? Then I found the Terrence Higgins Trust. That was part of saving me. I used their direct number, then went on to their newly diagnosed group, which really, really helped me. I met people in the same situation as me – people like Roland. I began to understand that it wasn't just me going through this.

We learned how to live a normal life. What the medications do, how to keep track of medication, the support that's out there. Who do I need to tell, what do I need to tell –you've got to be 100% sure when you tell someone, because you can never untell them.

After the newly diagnosed group, I decided to volunteer with THT and I'm still volunteering there today. I've done public speaking for THT on their behalf, working in campaigns, and actually, what has happened now is, from what my mum said, that I've turned my life around and although I would never wish HIV on anyone, it's actually changed my life for the better. I have a clear goal, which is to educate people so nobody has to be in the position that I was – for them to want to take their own life.

I also go to schools and businesses and I tell them my story, very openly, and let them ask any questions they want about it. I go into youth groups. I work for another charity called CHIVA – The Children's HIV Association – where I work at their summer camps in the summer, giving pastoral care to children living with HIV.

Mine and James's relationship has survived; something that not many do. We now own a flat together and we're getting married next June. It's better than it ever has been.

So there is the occasional thing like that, but I'm still in the process of telling people and the goal is to tell most of the people in our lives by next year. We don't want a room full of people at our wedding that don't know about us.

*

I'm in the process of wondering how to tell my employers about my HIV status. The nanny industry is very small, so if they reacted badly and told someone, I wouldn't be able to nanny in London again. I don't think it'll be a problem, but I'm not in a position to throw away my job just yet. I've battled for twelve years to work in an industry where men aren't appreciated for wanting to work with young children. So I have to pick the right time. I did tell my first employer as I am their children's godfather. They were fabulous, they've been a huge support, because I still see them quite a lot.

What I'm actually doing is slowly changing my career into HIV awareness permanently. I don't want to hide it from anyone important in my life. I want to be open, and I want to be proud of the achievements, and what I've overcome, and I can't do that when people I spend most of my life with don't know. So, that's why I want to tell my present employers.

I just want to make sure that nobody goes through what I've been through without support, and I want the stigma to be eradicated around HIV and for the government to take it seriously. I want sex education to be much clearer in schools and that people are more informed so they take responsibility for their own sex lives. It's really important that people like me don't have to hide away in the dark. It's a big goal but that is what I want to achieve.

The day I was diagnosed HIV positive was also the first night I slept on the streets of Camden.

SIMON HORVAT-MARCOVIC
AGE: 53
DATE OF DIAGNOSIS: 2 JULY 2015

Of all the things that happened to me in 2015, HIV was by no means the worst. Essentially my whole life imploded. I had two cancer scares, I lost my job, I was made homeless, I was diagnosed with three life-changing chronic illnesses, my thirteen-year relationship, including a nine-year civil partnership, came to an end. I was arrested and charged with drug possession. My mental health was such a mess I contemplated suicide twice. Not the happiest of years to put it mildly. You name it, it's been thrown at me, and guess what? I'm still here. Sheer bloody-mindedness I think. And I intend to be around a long time.

Some of this I put down to my heritage. My father is Austrian, his father was Yugoslavian and his father was Hungarian. So I come from good European stock. My grandmother was deported – we have photographs and news clippings of her being escorted across the tarmac by police officers at Croydon (the then London Airport). There were questions in the Houses of Parliament about it. She was stateless due to the war. She had a lot to deal with bringing up five children alone.

My maternal grandfather was in the RAF. He had got through the war as a navigator and pilot, then in 1948 he was one of the thirty-nine British Airmen to die in the Berlin Airlift. My maternal grandmother was the first civilian woman to cross the Iron Curtain, as his plane had crashed in the Russian sector.

My sister is a year younger than me and my brother eight years younger. My parents separated and divorced when I was thirteen. So we moved back to Stratford-upon-Avon from Yorkshire. My mother had to go out to work to support us, so I would come home from school and cook dinner for a family of four. My sister did the washing up. So basically my childhood stopped at that age.

I went to Stratford High School and then Further Education College. Being dyslexic I passed my exams but nothing majorly academic. My first job out of college came about out of nepotism. My aunt and father worked for a manufacturing jeweller as sales reps and so I became a rep with a huge territory, from the borders of Scotland down to Sutton in Surrey. I then moved into the Civil Service, firstly in the School Health Department then on to the Inland Revenue. This was followed by me becoming a Parliamentary Election agent, working in various parts of the UK. But this was not a secure income so I moved into retail management for a number of well-known high street stores, including working as a sales manager in the toy department of Harrods.

During my time working in Birmingham, I took up nightclub management duties as a second job in the Nightingale club, the biggest gay-owned club in the country. This came to an end when my main job took me to London. In 2010 my branch manager role had to be redeployed with a subsequent 46% pay cut. Luckily friends of mine who were DJ's and club owners needed a club manager. So during the day I would work my main job, then at night I would take on my nightclub manager duties, working an average ninety-eight-hour week at the age of forty-eight.

I was eventually hired by an extremely rich couple in St John's Wood as an estate manager, PA and driver. All was going well until my health started to take a downturn. This was the beginning of 2015. I thought I had cancer. When you get that emergency two-week hospital referral it scares you. I was really sick, in and out of hospital. Finally, I was made redundant because my boss couldn't rely on me being around. At the beginning of May my landlord informed me he was selling the flat I had lived in for sixteen years. So I was going to be homeless.

On the 2 July I was diagnosed as being HIV positive, following my usual quarterly sexual health screening. No wonder I was feeling so ill. They called me back, which wasn't an issue for me as I had had these tests for years. So I walked into the health advisors' room and I said, "Before you say anything, you're going to tell me I'm HIV positive." This was based on all the crap that was being thrown in my direction over the previous six months. The actual diagnosis wasn't an issue for me, as I have friends who have been positive for years. I didn't know as much then as I do now but it was the least of my worries, because it wasn't cancer, although I did get a second scare later that year which turned out to be a false alarm. At the time of my diagnosis I was sofa surfing, but that night I had no place to go. So the day I was diagnosed HIV positive was also the first night I slept on the streets of Camden.

I had a very low viral load and a very high CD4 count. Thanks to a great HIV consultant I was allowed to start medication straight away. Within one month I was undetectable. And have remained so.

Now I had had the discussions about how I contracted HIV. I worked out there were twenty-five guys in four different continents that I had been with between my sexual health screenings in February 2015 and July 2015. That's not saying it was unsafe or anything like that, but I decided I would phone every single one. And the first thing they mostly said was not "I had better get tested" it was more a matter of "Are you OK?" (as in me). That knocked me for six. The point is younger people today are more aware that it's chronic and not a killer, unless you don't take the medication or if there are complications.

To turn the clocks back a couple of months, while I was sofa surfing, the police turned up to my friend's flat at 4am as he had an outstanding bench warrant due to unpaid council tax. As he answered the door just in his boxer shorts, they brought him back into the flat to dress. Four police officers found me naked in bed, except for a big smile. There were recreational drugs in the flat so we were both arrested. For eight years I had been the Chair of my local Safer

Neighbourhoods' Panel, I had been an Independent Custody Visitor for five years and been on police committees. I was even having meetings in New Scotland Yard. Obviously that all disappeared overnight. I was handcuffed, shoved in the back of a police van, taken to a police cell, strip searched by two officers then arrested. I thought I'd be cautioned but I was prosecuted. I knew the arrest procedure. I asked for a copy of PACE and was told, "You're the first person to ask for that." It's the most boring book ever, but the point is that I asked for it, because it was my right to do so. Well that's just like me. Funny thing was, my keys were on a Metropolitan Police lanyard, which I thought was amusing as they sealed my possessions in the evidence bag. I was convicted for possession of Class A, Class B and Class C drugs. I was fined and given a twelve-month conditional discharge.

When I went back to the clinic following my court appearance I was informed that they had also screened me for Hepatitis C; they actually went back to two previous sexual health screenings. They wanted me to get my HIV medication regime working well before they would try to treat my Hep C but for me the problem was I had been bleeding for seven months due to my ulcerative colitis. I felt like a walking biohazard. They said I had had it from November 2014, which explained all the tiredness etc. So I had to contact the same twenty-five guys a second time to inform them.

I was hoping to start a new relationship with an Asian guy, but he said he couldn't take the pressure, because there was so much going on in my shambolic life. He wanted me to be the strong person, as I was twice his age, and he couldn't do it. I completely broke down. I couldn't take it anymore. I decided I'd put my world in order and I said my goodbyes via Facebook. I was heading home to my old flat to sort out a few things. I didn't want to embarrass my mother in what might be found after my death. I planned to kill myself using large amounts of recreational drugs. As I got to Kentish Town West

Overground station, the phone rang. It was my friend (the DJ) who had just had a liver transplant; he knew I was becoming homeless that week, and he wanted to make sure I was OK.

So, instead of turning left towards my old flat, I turned right and went to see my friend in his ICU ward. After that I realised life was worth living. A few months after his transplant there were complications and he passed away. At his funeral I went up to his twenty-one-year-old son and said "Your dad saved my life."

I was still homeless that autumn, and by Christmas I was in a crisis hostel in Highbury Grove. Normally it's meant to be a two-week stay, but I ended up there for four weeks. I was so frustrated by the housing allocation system that I actually threatened to bite the housing officer then kill myself, naming him in my suicide note. It was at this point I was escorted out of Camden Council offices by two huge bouncers. It resulted in the Crisis Team stepping in and starting to get things sorted. After living in a homeless hostel in Limehouse for nine months I was offered a small studio flat with a private landlord. For over a year I had no income, then finally was put on ESA at £73 per week. The flat I was offered had a £41 per week shortfall after my housing benefit, leaving me with £32 a week for all my expenses, food, travel and utilities. Then on Boxing Day I received a letter from Camden Council that I was being benefit-capped, leaving me a shortfall of £80 per week on my rent, to come out of my £73. But at least I had a place to live.

I received help from a Positively UK benefits advisor, who helped me go through the complex procedure for Personal Independent Payments (PiP), enabling me to get enhanced daily living allowance and enhanced mobility allowance. Once you get PiP, doors open. The cap disappears and due to my disability I got a Freedom Pass to use on the transport system in London.

A lot more happened to me but as I say, "Nothing's going to kill me, apart from me." I have depression and other mental and physical health issues. People always say "Be positive, be positive", then I became positive as in HIV positive, and that's fine. I now believe that I'm actually going to live longer and healthier now than I would've done without my diagnosis.

High blood pressure, high cholesterol, sciatica, ulcerative colitis are a few of the things wrong with me, but if I hadn't been positive they wouldn't have tested me for everything else. I was eventually treated for Hepatitis C. It was really heavy going, but after a few short weeks of treatment at the cost of £39,000 it was cleared. The only problem I have is the really scary knowledge that if I get reinfected they won't treat me, as you only get one hit with the new drugs.

I am trying to get fit, and also dealing with really bad tooth problems due to my not having money for food to eat whilst homeless and due to my ulcerative colitis. I knew I was losing blood, I'm now anaemic but I was also losing calcium.

I have good weeks and bad like most people. I realised one week I hadn't spoken to a human in over a week. The only thing I spoke with was my Google Home – Hey Google. I also realised if you set long-term goals, you fall flat on your face, so I deal with short and medium-term goals. I am not going to put myself under too much pressure, I have somewhere to live and it's paid for. I don't have a huge amount of money to live on but it's enough. Remember I survived for a year with no income, so I make do.

I take full responsibility for everything that happened to me. I wasn't held prisoner. It was nobody else's fault. Hopefully they will sort out my long-term physical pain. But my mental health will be a long journey. I have good days and bad days. I was diagnosed with reactive depression with anxiety. Well if you think about it, shit happens – that's why you feel shit!

I lived my life publicly on Facebook, my Hep C, my

homelessness, mental health problems, drug issues, the lot, but the one issue I didn't disclose was my being positive. With that declaration you've got to think who's getting what out of it? Do they need to know and if they need to, why? Does it harm you or them?

During Pride 2016 I was with Positively UK. Actually that's where I came out to the whole world, because I was marching under the banner 'Proudly Undetectable' I changed my profile picture of me wearing a t-shirt with it on, I literally wore the t-shirt. At Pride 2017 I marched with the Terrence Higgins Trust where they launched their #CAN'T PASS IT ON campaign.

I have trained to be a peer mentor with Positively UK and am undergoing training with THT to be part of their Positive Voices programme, where I will go in to schools and work places and share my experiences of being HIV positive.

What I'm missing is a relationship. I miss a cuddle, I miss somebody holding me. Sex is easy, extremely so. I am even doing a group counselling programme at THT about losing control, basically to do with sex, drugs and dating apps. What I am trying to do is give myself the tools to ensure I don't fall back into my old ways. I don't want to get Hep C again, and the best way to contract that is by going back to the chemsex parties. I can't say that I will steer clear of recreational drugs in the future. But they were never the focus, more like the icing on the cake. At the Newly Diagnosed workshop I did with Positively UK back in August 2015, there were fourteen guys there. I was the oldest, I had taken the most drugs and I was the most promiscuous one there. I tried to pick up three of the guys in the workshop. I'm very brash, I'm very forward, I'm loud but it's a shell of course. I now steer clear of most things, I still have fun occasionally but I am not how I used to be, I try to keep a balance.

I wear my status on my sleeve. It's there for all to see. Now that I can't pass it on, its easier to explain about Undetectable is

Untransmittable, #CAN'T PASS IT ON. I do declare and if they don't like it, it's their problem not mine.

You know we are the fifth richest country in the world, but the housing and homeless issues we are facing are shocking. It's not the same as it used to be, when I moved to London in 1998. The homeless were battling drink and drug problems, now its families, the young, everyone really. While I was sofa surfing I would be stopped by people begging on the streets. Sometimes I would tell them all that was going on in my life and they would apologise and move on. But I remember one guy who looked really down on his luck. I had just come from one of my numerous medical appointments and was walking from the Royal Free Hospital back to my Limehouse homeless hostel as I didn't have money for public transport. I had two pound coins in my pocket and that was to last me the rest of the week. I said to him I only had two pound coins, but I said he should have one if it bought him a loaf of bread, he'd get something to eat.

So yeah that's my outlook on life. It's to give something back. If you can do something and you can make one person's life a little easier, that's a good thing and in the process I'll get better.

What would I do differently? To be honest, the point is at least we know better, but we're human and we're fallible. I've had a lot of experience, a lot of life. If I can prove to someone that it's not worthless, it's not a waste of time, fight back, then great. The system is geared against you and it's crap, but there are ways and means and there are people out there to help. Make sure you speak to somebody. Part of joining the peer mentor group at Positively UK is that we want to make sure that everybody who is positive can get access to a peer mentor. It is so much better when you're talking to a person that has walked in your shoes. We've done the same journey, we're just a bit further down the road, that's all.

AFTERWORD

More than 102,000 people are currently (late 2017) living with HIV in the UK. In this book you have read only fourteen of our stories. Each story is exceptional and unique but linked by a common thread. There are so many other stories out there still to be told. Not only of people who are managing, somehow, an HIV diagnosis, and the impact it has had on their lives, but of all those people who too are managing a life-changing diagnosis of any kind.

This book is dedicated to them.

PRAISE FOR *RIPPLES FROM THE EDGE OF LIFE*

Roland captures his powerful, personal story, and the stories of those who stood alongside him on the way in a book that engages and inspires in equal measure.

Grant Sugden, Chief Executive, Waverley Care, www.waverleycare.org/

Ripples from the Edge of Life is an absorbing and moving testament to real lives lived, and a tribute to lives lost, in a particular time and place in the story of HIV.

There is no other diagnosis quite like HIV. It is easy to say that these days it is a health condition that can be managed very effectively with medication, and so it is, for very many people. But living with HIV is not just about medicine. A diagnosis brings with it a complex web of feelings, social attitudes and beliefs both for the person directly affected and for everyone in their lives. Everybody has a view about what it means to be HIV positive and sadly, there is no other condition that has the same level of stigma associated with it.

As well as telling his own story of how his life changed irrevocably on September 1st 2006, and the rippling consequences of that for everyone in his life, Roland draws together the experiences of others who have faced the same diagnosis across the three decades in which we have been responding to HIV in the UK.

The chapters are filled with eloquent voices that tell us how it is to live with HIV, with all the ups and downs, the pluses and minuses. All experiences are reflected in these pages and these are voices that deserve to be heard.

Siobhán Lanigan, CEO, The Food Chain, www.foodchain.org.uk/

It's been 25 years since GMFA (Gay Men Fighting AIDS) was formed. In 1992, a group of gay men got together and decided that not enough was being done to tackle HIV and AIDS in the gay community. Back then we lived in a very different world, and there was no functional medication. When gay men were diagnosed with HIV, many were told to start planning for their deaths. This was the stark reality in 1992.

Many of the founding members of GMFA lived through some of the toughest times our community has ever seen. Others never got to see past the first few years of GMFA. It was a difficult time and as members of GMFA died, others stepped in to fill the void. Gay men knew that they were living in an era where if they didn't look after each other, no one else would. GMFA saved a lot of lives in the early years. Today, many of these men are leading normal, healthy and happy lives.

We must never forget where we have come from and we must never lose focus on what we are trying to achieve. I think this book does exactly that. Behind every diagnosis is a human being who has to live with the virus. Being told you are living with HIV is life changing. Everything you knew before has changed forever. You not only have to live with the virus, you also have to live with society and the stigma it places on people living with HIV. And that is tough.

Over 100,000 people in the UK are living with HIV. That's 100,000 people who are living, breathing and existing in a world where people forget where we have come from. These 100,000 people are here today because we fought a battle against HIV and AIDS – and although the battle isn't over, we are heading in the right direction.

What this book does is shine a light on some of the people battling through life with HIV. These honest, life-changing stories are prime examples of the true faces of HIV. Each story made me think about the person, not the virus. It brought humanity to all the work we at GMFA are trying to do. Humanity is the key to ending HIV and HIV stigma.

Roland has produced a wonderful book. These stories will touch your heart and enrage your mind. They remind me of what we all need to do to end HIV once and for all. I hope that after you read this book you raise a glass to all those we have lost to HIV and AIDS since the early 1980s and then drink to the thousands of people in the UK who are not only surviving but thriving while living a healthy, normal life. Our battle against HIV isn't over yet, but if we all come together we can end HIV.

Ian Howley, CEO, GMFA, www.gmfa.org.uk/

The accounts presented in this book are all too familiar to many of us within the National Long-Term Survivors Group (NLTSG). We often hear from those more recently diagnosed positive that they take great solace from those who have gone through the worst of it.

If this book does nothing but assist in breaking down the stigma of a positive diagnosis then it will have performed a powerful task.

Even within the group, many take inspiration from those who have been through it, and others get to realise that they are not alone. If the ripples from these powerful accounts do no more than to get others to become a little more understanding and less judgemental, then it will have achieved its goal. For the majority now, it is just a chronic condition, but it may well also impact many aspects of your life.

Tremaine Cornish, Treasurer, NLTSG, www.nltsg.org.uk/

Ripples gives a unique insight into the emotional rollercoaster of an HIV diagnosis and its lifelong impact. Reading the personal experiences was haunting and reinforced the importance of having flexible HIV support services to meet the differing needs of each person and challenged the assumption that one size fits all. Definitely one of my top-recommended reads.

Steph Mallas, CEO. George House Trust, Manchester, ght.org.uk/

I was gripped from the first moment by Roland Chesters' autobiography, *Ripples*. As one who remembers the government's tombstone ads of the 1980s and whose sexual behaviours were undoubtedly affected by them, I was only too pleased to be asked to provide some comment. Roland provides glimpses into his early life, which provide context and allow us to connect with him early on in the book. This carries the readers through because we have come to care about him and what happens to him along the way. His subtle use of humour to deal with the impact of his HIV diagnosis and people's responses to that provides a pendulum of light and shade throughout. The inclusion of other HIV narratives from both men and women provides a really rounded view of people's experiences. Roland's book is many things – an illness narrative, a potted history of HIV, a handbook if you are diagnosed, a love story and, most importantly, a challenge to the reduced but continued stigma surrounding this condition.

Dr Ava Easton, Chief Executive, The Encephalitis Society, www. encephalitis.info/Default.aspx

Lightning Source UK Ltd.
Milton Keynes UK
UKHW010429090419
340717UK00001B/306/P

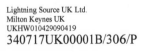

9 781781 327098